Michael Lichtenauer

Secretome of apoptotic cells and myocardial infarction

Michael Lichtenauer

Secretome of apoptotic cells and myocardial infarction

Ways of cardioprotection after myocardial infarction by paracrine factors

Südwestdeutscher Verlag für Hochschulschriften

Impressum/Imprint (nur für Deutschland/only for Germany)
Bibliografische Information der Deutschen Nationalbibliothek: Die Deutsche Nationalbibliothek verzeichnet diese Publikation in der Deutschen Nationalbibliografie; detaillierte bibliografische Daten sind im Internet über http://dnb.d-nb.de abrufbar.
Alle in diesem Buch genannten Marken und Produktnamen unterliegen warenzeichen-, marken- oder patentrechtlichem Schutz bzw. sind Warenzeichen oder eingetragene Warenzeichen der jeweiligen Inhaber. Die Wiedergabe von Marken, Produktnamen, Gebrauchsnamen, Handelsnamen, Warenbezeichnungen u.s.w. in diesem Werk berechtigt auch ohne besondere Kennzeichnung nicht zu der Annahme, dass solche Namen im Sinne der Warenzeichen- und Markenschutzgesetzgebung als frei zu betrachten wären und daher von jedermann benutzt werden dürften.

Coverbild: www.ingimage.com

Verlag: Südwestdeutscher Verlag für Hochschulschriften GmbH & Co. KG
Heinrich-Böcking-Str. 6-8, 66121 Saarbrücken, Deutschland
Telefon +49 681 37 20 271-1, Telefax +49 681 37 20 271-0
Email: info@svh-verlag.de

Approved by: Wien, Medizinische Universität Wien, Dissertation, 2011

Herstellung in Deutschland:
Schaltungsdienst Lange o.H.G., Berlin
Books on Demand GmbH, Norderstedt
Reha GmbH, Saarbrücken
Amazon Distribution GmbH, Leipzig
ISBN: 978-3-8381-3186-3

Imprint (only for USA, GB)
Bibliographic information published by the Deutsche Nationalbibliothek: The Deutsche Nationalbibliothek lists this publication in the Deutsche Nationalbibliografie; detailed bibliographic data are available in the Internet at http://dnb.d-nb.de.
Any brand names and product names mentioned in this book are subject to trademark, brand or patent protection and are trademarks or registered trademarks of their respective holders. The use of brand names, product names, common names, trade names, product descriptions etc. even without a particular marking in this works is in no way to be construed to mean that such names may be regarded as unrestricted in respect of trademark and brand protection legislation and could thus be used by anyone.

Cover image: www.ingimage.com

Publisher: Südwestdeutscher Verlag für Hochschulschriften GmbH & Co. KG
Heinrich-Böcking-Str. 6-8, 66121 Saarbrücken, Germany
Phone +49 681 37 20 271-1, Fax +49 681 37 20 271-0
Email: info@svh-verlag.de

Printed in the U.S.A.
Printed in the U.K. by (see last page)
ISBN: 978-3-8381-3186-3

Copyright © 2012 by the author and Südwestdeutscher Verlag für Hochschulschriften GmbH & Co. KG and licensors
All rights reserved. Saarbrücken 2012

"Hic locus est ubi mors gaudet succurrere vitae"
(This is the place where death delights to help the living)

Giovanni Battista Morgagni (1682 – 1771)

Inscription at the Institute of Anatomy, Medical University Vienna

DANKSAGUNG

Ich möchte mich bei all jenen bedanken, die mich bei der Durchführung und der Verfassung dieser Arbeit sowohl fachlich als auch persönlich unterstützt haben.

Ganz besonders danken möchte ich meinen Eltern Ingrid und Heinz, die mir nicht nur das Studium der Humanmedizin ermöglicht haben, sondern mich auch während meines PhD Studiums in allen erdenklichen Lebenslagen unterstützt haben.

Die Resultate dieser Studie wurden im Rahmen mehrerer internationaler und nationaler Kongresse präsentiert, u.a. bei der Jahrestagung der International Society for Heart and Lung Transplantation (ISHLT 2011) in San Diego 2011 und beim Kongress der European Society for Cardiology (ESC) in Stockholm (2010) bzw. Paris (2011).
Im Rahmen der Jahrestagung der Österreichischen Kardiologischen Gesellschaft (ÖKG) in Salzburg erhielt die dieser Arbeit zugrundeliegende Publikation den österreichischen Kardiologenpreis 2011 (1. Platz Basic Science).

Die beiden zu dieser Arbeit gehörigen Originalarbeiten wurden im Journal *Basic Research in Cardiology* publiziert. Die vollständigen Publikationen finden sich im Anhang am Ende dieser Dissertation.

Table of Contents

Zusammenfassung...	6
Abstract...	8
Introduction...	10
Stem Cell Therapies for Acute Myocardial Infarction........................	10
The Dying Stem Cell Hypothesis...	11
Apoptotic Cell Therapy for AMI..	12
The Paracrine Paradigm..	16
Aims of the study..	17
Materials and Methods..	19
Descriptions of proceedings investigating the cardioprotective properties of apoptotic PBMC..	19
Acquisition of syngeneic rat PBMC suspensions for *in vivo* experiments..	19
Induction of acute myocardial infarction in male Sprague-Dawley rats...	20
Histological and immunohistological evaluations.......................	20
Evaluation of cardiac function by echocardiography six weeks after induction of myocardial infarction...	21
Separation of human PBMC for *in vitro* experiments..................	22
Cell culture of human fibroblasts exposed to supernatants of apoptotic PBMC, RNA isolation and cDNA preparation.............	22
Quantitative real time polymerase chain reaction (RT-PCR)......	23
Semi-quantitative evaluation of cytokines and growth factors secreted by apoptotic PBMC by means of membrane arrays....	24
Descriptions of proceedings investigating the cardioprotective properties of cell culture supernatants of apoptotic PBMC (APOSEC)..	25
Production of $APOSEC^H$, $APOSEC^R$ and $APOSEC^P$ – Supernatants derived from irradiated apoptotic PBMC.............	25
Membrane array and ELISA analysis of cytokines and growth factors in $APOSEC^H$...	26
Rat AMI model and $APOSEC^R$ treatment.................................	27
Histological and immunohistological analysis and determination of myocardial infarction size by planimetry............................	27
Enzymatic digestion of infarcted myocardium and flow cytometric analysis..	28
Assessment of cardiac function by means of echocardiography.	28

Large animal AMI model..	28
In situ viability staining using tetrazolium chloride...................	30
Measurement of Troponin I levels after AMI...........................	30
Determination of cardiac functional parameters after AMI by magnetic resonance imaging (MRI)...	31
Cell culture of primary human cardiomyocytes and immunoblot analysis...	31
Statistical methods...	32

Results... 33

Results of experiments investigating the cardioprotective properties of apoptotic PBMC... 33

Histological analysis of cardiac specimens obtained three days after AMI...	33
Immunohistological staining for CD68, c-kit and VEGF-R2..........	34
Histological evaluation six weeks after LAD ligation...................	36
Assessment of cardiac function by echocardiography................	38
Analysis of the composition of left ventricular scar tissue six weeks after AMI...	38
Different secretion patterns of cytokines, chemokines and growth factors in apoptotic cells...	42

Results of experiments investigating the cardioprotective properties of supernatants obtained from apoptotic PBMC............... 46

Analysis of soluble factors detectable in cell culture supernatants of irradiated human PBMC (termed APOSEC^H).....	46
Up-regulation of anti-apoptotic and cytoprotective factors by supernatants of apoptotic cells..	50
APOSEC treatment in a rat model of AMI.................................	55
Assessment of cardiac function by means of echocardiography..	61
Large animal AMI model...	63
Cardiac MRI evaluation 3 and 30 days after AMI......................	68
BARI score evaluations..	69

Discussion..	70
Conclusion..	75
References..	76

Zusammenfassung

Der akute Myokardinfarkt gefolgt von linksventrikulärem Remodelling ist eine der Hauptursachen für die chronische Herzinsuffizienz in der westlichen Welt. Vorangegangene Untersuchungen zeigten, dass die Injektion apoptotischer Zellen im Tiermodell des Herzinfarkts die Infarktgröße signifikant reduzieren, die linksventrikuläre Funktion erhalten und das Einwandern regenerativer Zellpopulationen in die Ischämiezone fördern konnte. Ziel dieser Studie war, die diesen Effekten zugrundeliegenden Mechanismen zu entschlüsseln. Ein besonderes Augenmerk wurde auf die Rolle parakriner Faktoren, die von apoptotischen Zellen sezerniert werden, gelegt.

Suspensionen apoptotischer Zellen wurden in einem Rattenmodell des akuten Herzinfarkts einerseits intravenös als auch intramyokardial injiziert. Morphologische und funktionelle Analysen wurden mittels Histologie, Planimetrie und Echokardiographie durchgeführt.
Die kardioprotektiven Eigenschaften von Zellkulturüberständen apoptotischer Zellen wurden in einem weiteren Rattenmodell des akuten Herzinfarkts mittels permanenter Gefäßligatur und ebenfalls in einem Großtiermodell mit anschließender Reperfusion evaluiert.

Planimetrische und echokardiografische Analysen zeigten eine signifikante Reduktion der Infarktgröße mit geringeren Anzeichen von linksventrikulärer Dilatation und eine verbesserte linksventrikuläre Funktion in Tieren, denen Suspensionen apoptotischer Zeller injiziert wurden. In einer histologischen Auswertung zeigte sich, dass das kardiale Narbengewebe von therapierten Tieren eine weit höhere Akkumulation von elastischen Fasern aufwies.
Durch die ausschließliche Verabreichung von Zellkulturüberständen apoptotischer Zellen konnte ebenfalls sowohl im Kleintier- als auch im Großtiermodell eine Reduktion der Infarktgröße und eine Verbesserung kardialer Funktionsparameter erzielt werden. *In vitro* Assays zeigten, dass humane Kardiomyozyten, die mit Zellkulturüberständen apoptotischer Zellen inkubiert wurden, eine Hochregulierung

von anti-apoptotischen Mediatoren (Bcl-2, BAG1) und eine Aktivierung von kardioprotektiven Signalkaskaden (u.a. Akt, Erk1/2, CREB) zeigten.

Diese Daten zeigen, dass die Verabreichung von apoptotischen Zellen beziehungsweise deren Zellkulturüberständen, zytoprotektive Signalwege in Kardiomyozyten induzieren und so den Infarktschaden reduzieren kann.

Abstract

Heart failure developing after acute myocardial ischaemia is a major cause of morbidity and mortality in the western world. In our previous study we showed that intravenous injection of apoptotic peripheral blood mononuclear cell (PBMC) suspensions preserved cardiac function in a rat acute myocardial infarction (AMI) model. Based on these results, we sought to investigate other ways of cell administration and analysed the composition of the fibrotic scar tissue. Moreover, we sought to study the effect of soluble factors secreted by apoptotic PBMC on ventricular remodelling after AMI.

Cell suspensions of apoptotic PBMC were injected intravenously (IV) or intramyocardially (IM) after experimental AMI in rats. The administration of cell culture medium or viable PBMC served as controls. To study the effects of paracrine factors secreted by apoptotic cells, supernatants of irradiated PBMC were collected and injected intravenously after myocardial infarction in an experimental AMI rat model and in a porcine closed chest reperfused AMI model.

Rats injected with suspensions of apoptotic PBMC (either intravenously or intramyocardially) evidenced a significant reduction of infarct dimensions and preservation of cardiac function. Histology showed that the ratio of elastic and collagenous fibres within the scar tissue was altered in a favourable fashion in rats injected with apoptotic cells compared to controls.

The administration of supernatants of apoptotic PBMC resulted in a reduction of myocardial scar tissue formation in both the rat and the porcine model. In the large animal reperfused AMI model higher values of ejection fraction (57.0% vs. 40.5%, p<0.01), a better cardiac output (4.0 vs. 2.4 l/min., p<0.001) and a reduced extent of infarction size (12.6% vs. 6.9%, p<0.02) were found. *In vitro* experiments showed that exposure of primary human cardiac myocytes with paracrine factors secreted by apoptotic PBMC induced the activation of pro-survival signalling-cascades (AKT, Erk1/2, CREB) and increased anti-apoptotic gene products (Bcl-2, BAG1).

Intravenous and intramyocardial injection of apoptotic cell suspensions preserved left ventricular function and altered the composition of cardiac scar tissue with increased expression of elastic fibres. Intravenous infusion of cell culture supernatants of apoptotic PBMC attenuated myocardial remodelling in both experimental AMI animal models.

Introduction

Stem Cell Therapies for Acute Myocardial Infarction

New treatment strategies and early reperfusion within a narrow time window has significantly reduced the mortality following acute myocardial infarction (AMI). However, ischaemic heart failure secondary to the initial event still remains widely prevalent and represents an increasing economic burden in the western world [1].

Great expectations emerged in the scientific world when Orlic *et al.* discovered in 2001 that the injection of bone marrow stem cells expressing the marker c-kit lead to the regeneration of myocardial tissue and reduced ventricular remodelling after AMI [2]. These findings were supported by an abundance of experimental studies published shortly after [3-5]. Over the following years many randomized controlled clinical trials were implemented in order to investigate whether injection of autologous stem cells supports healing processes after AMI or can even regenerate viable myocardium.

One of the largest clinical trials (the REPAIR-AMI trial) evaluating regenerative effects of bone marrow cells in patients after AMI was published in 2006 [6]. The REPAIR-AMI investigators showed that in patients being injected with autologous bone marrow derived progenitor cells, the global left ventricular ejection fraction (EF) was improved significantly after four months and mortality was reduced within the first year.

However, the ASTAMI trial failed to show or prove any beneficial effects of stem administration after AMI [7]. The authors speculated that the way of cell administration (i.e. by intracoronary delivery) has many limitations, only a small percentage of the injected cells might remain in the ischaemic heart and a further large proportion of transplanted cells might die within the next few days [8, 9].

The BOOST study was the clinical trial investigating cardiac cell therapy after AMI with the longest follow-up period. Even though initial results were very convincing showing a significant improvement of EF after six months of follow-up, results failed to show significance after 18 months and to an even lesser extent after 61 months [10-12].

In order to further evaluate these controversial results meta-analysis were conducted. Some suggested that cell therapy after AMI might improve EF but it does not prevent ventricular remodelling whereas others stated that there is not enough evidence to support the clinical application of stem cell therapy after AMI [13, 14]. However, the mechanistic principles of cardiac stem cell therapy still remain unclear as many other interactions such as pro-angiogenic effects, immunomodulation or paracrine signalling might be involved.

The Dying Stem Cell Hypothesis

Inflammation due to myocardial necrosis after ischaemia is an integral part in the pathophysiology of cellular responses after AMI. These inflammatory reactions in the ischaemic myocardium contribute to the detrimental processes after AMI subsequently leading to loss of further cardiomyocytes and to ventricular remodelling. Thum et al. stated in their hypothesis published in 2005 that immunomodulatory signals induced by transplanted apoptotic stem cells might be responsible for the (mildly) beneficial effects seen in clinical trials [15]. In these trials, the proportion of cells already undergoing apoptosis ranged around 5 to 25 percent [10, 16-18]. The authors assumed that necrosis of cardiomyocytes within the ischaemic myocardium plays the predominant part in triggering pro-inflammatory signals in the cellular microenvironment. They proposed that the improvement in cardiac function seen after stem cells administration might be explained by the modulatory interactions of local immune cells in response to transplanted cells undergoing apoptosis. It was shown that in contrast to necrotic cells, apoptotic cells can inhibit inflammatory reactions. This phenomenon was extensively covered by the work of Fadok et al. [19, 20].

It was shown previously that the recognition of apoptotic particles by phagocytic cells, such as macrophages is mediated via interaction of phosphatidylserine receptors. This interaction requires exposure of phosphatidylserine, which usually is only found on the inner leaflet of the plasma membrane of every cell, to flip to the outer surface of the apoptotic cell. They further argued that the ingestion of apoptotic cells by macrophages leads to the expression of the anti-inflammatory cytokines, such as interleukin-10 (IL-10) and transforming growth factor beta (TGF-beta).

In the pro-inflammatory microenvironment of necrotic tissues the increased expression of anti-inflammatory cytokines counteracting the signaling of pro-inflammatory mediators such as tumor necrosis factor alpha (TNF-alpha), interleukin-1 beta (IL-1beta) and interleukin-6 (IL-6) might result in an accelerated resolution of detrimental inflammatory processes after AMI and might improve reparative effects.
The group of Fadok furthermore showed conclusively that phagocytes that have ingested apoptotic but not necrotic cells respond by a change of the secretion pattern of many pro-survival growth factors such as vascular endothelial growth factor (VEGF) or hepatocyte growth factor (HGF). These factors play a major role in conferring cytoprotective signals to neighboring cells by up-regulation of the anti-apoptotic protein Bcl-2, via phosphatidylinositol 3-kinase (PI3K) and triggering of the AKT signal transduction pathway [21].

Apoptotic Cell Therapy for AMI

In our previous study we tried to verify the hypothesis by Thum *et al.* [15] using *in vitro* and *in vivo* experiments. In order to implement the findings of Fadok *et al.* [19-21] into Thum's hypothesis, we tested the immunosuppressive or immunomodulatory effects of apoptotic cells in *in vitro* assays and their cardioprotective potential in a rat model of AMI.

We could show that the addition of irradiated apoptotic peripheral blood mononuclear cells (PBMC) reduced the secretion of the pro-inflammatory cytokines Interleukin-1beta (IL-1beta) and Interleukin-6 (IL-6) in an *in vitro* assay of LPS (bacterial lipopolysaccharide) stimulated cell cultures of monocytes and PBMC. Similar effects were also observed in mixed-lymphocyte reaction assays [22].

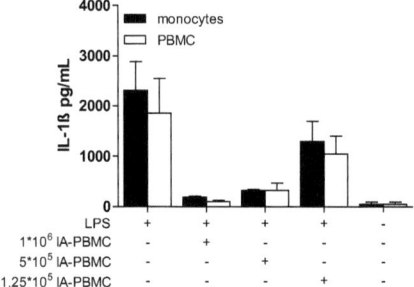 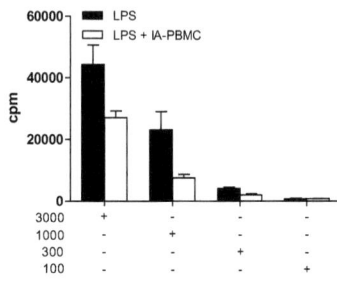

Figure 1 Co-incubation of LPS stimulated monocytes and PBMC with irradiated apoptotic PBMC suspensions reduced the secretory capacity of IL-1beta. Concomitantly, the addition of irradiated apoptotic PBMC to mixed-lymphocyte reactions decreased cell proliferation as indicated by less counts per minute (cpm)[22].

In the *in vivo* part of our previous study we injected syngeneic irradiated apoptotic PBMC suspensions in a rat model of AMI induced by ligation of the left anterior descending artery (LAD) via an intravenous route. We could show that the intravenous administration of irradiated apoptotic PBMC suspensions reduced infarct dimensions and scar formation six weeks after induction of AMI and also preserved ventricular function as evidenced by significantly improved values of ejection fraction (EF) and shortening fraction (SF). Moreover, higher numbers of cells staining positively for endothelial progenitor cell markers such as c-kit and Vascular endothelial growth factor receptor 2 (VEGF-R2) [23-25] were found within the cellular infiltrate in the ischaemic myocardium in animals injected with apoptotic cells. When evaluating cardiac tissue specimens, we also found higher numbers of macrophages in the ischaemic myocardium of treated animals compared to controls.

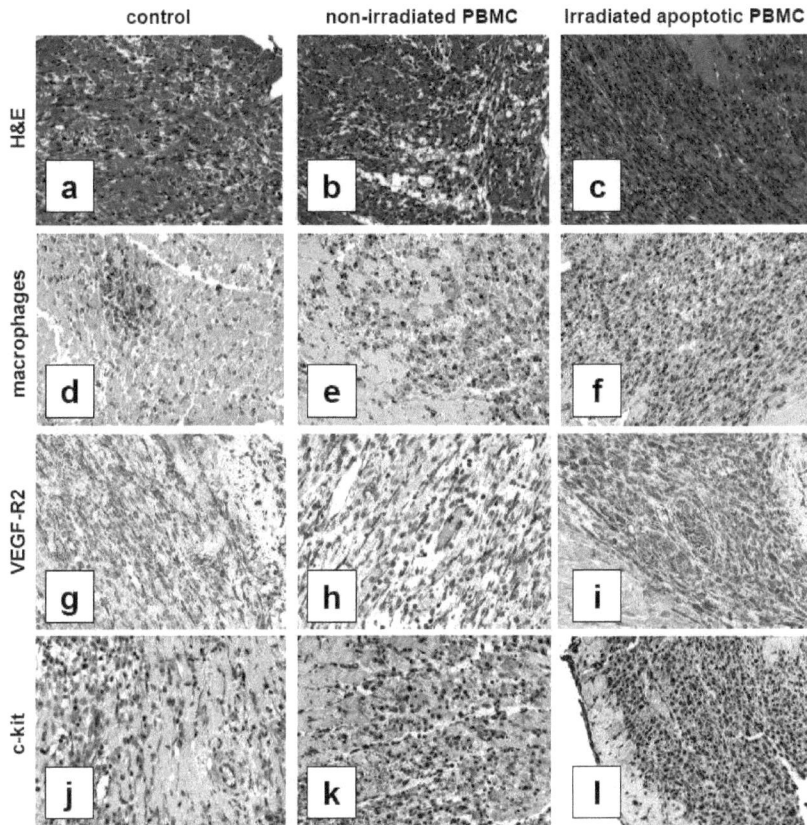

Figure 2 Tissue specimens stained with haematoxylin and eosin (H&E staining) evidenced that the cellular infiltrate was much denser in rats injected with apoptotic PBMC (c) compared to controls (a) and animals injected with non-irradiated viable cells (b). Moreover, higher numbers of macrophages and cells staining positively for VEGF-R2 and c-kit were found after injection of apoptotic PBMC following LAD ligation (f,i,l) compared to control groups (d,e,g,h,j,k)[22].

Six weeks after induction of AMI, hearts were explanted and infarct dimensions were calculated by means of planimetry. A significant reduction in infarct dimension was apparent in animals injected with irradiated apoptotic PBMC over controls and also over rats injected with non-irradiated viable cells.

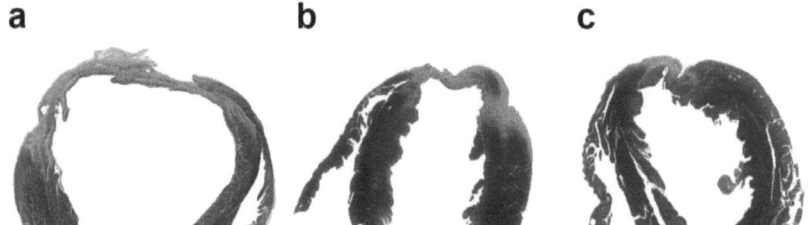

Figure 3 shows mid-ventricular sections of hearts explanted six weeks after induction of AMI. Large infarcts were common in the control group (a), a slight improvement was found in animals injected with viable cells (b) and the best outcome was observed in rats injected with irradiated apoptotic cells (c)[22].

Parameters of cardiac function were evaluated by means of echocardiography six weeks after AMI. Whereas both in controls as in animals injected with non-irradiated cells a significant loss of cardiac function was apparent compared to healthy rats (sham operated), functional parameters were almost completely preserved in animals with intravenous injection of irradiated apoptotic cells.

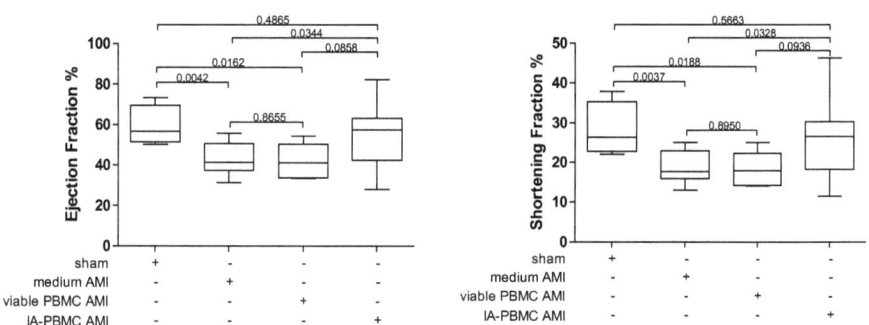

Figure 4 shows parameters of cardiac function (ejection fraction and shortening fraction) obtained six weeks after AMI by means of echocardiography. Rats injected with irradiated apoptotic cells presented a significant improvement of both ejection fraction and shortening fraction[22].

However, the exact mechanism how apoptotic cells reduced myocardial damage following AMI and preserved cardiac function still remained to be elucidated.

The Paracrine Paradigm

Over the last few years a new concept was developed in the field of regenerative therapies for AMI, namely that the main therapeutic effect seen in studies investigating stem cell therapy are conferred by paracrine factors that are secreted by the injected cells.

The first reports on this relatively new field of investigation date back to the year 2005, when Gnecchi *et al.* reported that the conditioned medium of mesenchymal stem cells stressed by incubation under hypoxic conditions significantly reduced the rate of cell death of adult rat ventricular cardiomyocytes caused by hypoxia [26]. The authors also tested their hypothesis in an *in vivo* model of AMI by permanent LAD ligation in a rat model and showed that the conditioned medium reduced the rate of apoptosis in the ischaemic myocardium. Moreover, infarct dimensions were reduced as well. The group of Gnecchi further proved their hypothesis in following studies and discussed their findings in many review articles [27-30].

In a sub-study conducted by the BOOST investigators, the regenerative effect of paracrine factors in human cardiac stem cell therapy was discussed for the first time [31]. In this study, the secretome of bone marrow derived cells and of peripheral blood cells was tested for its regenerative or cytoprotective effects in *in vitro* experiments, investigating coronary artery endothelial cell proliferation, migration, endothelial tube formation and aortic cell sprouting. Moreover, these cell culture supernatants protected rat cardiomyocytes from simulated ischaemia/reperfusion induced cell death in an *in vitro* model. Interestingly, both the supernatants of bone marrow cells and also of peripheral blood cells showed cytoprotective and regenerative effects in these assays with only marginal differences. The authors also compared the secretion pattern of the two cell types and found that bone marrow cells only produced slightly higher amounts of cytokines, chemokines and growth factors related to regenerative processes compared to peripheral blood cells.

These findings were supported by reports from the research group of Kalka *et al.*, they investigated the protective effects of endothelial progenitor cell (EPC) derived secretomes *in vitro* and in a rat model of hind limb ischaemia [32, 33]. These EPC derived secretomes reduced oxidative stress and the rate of apoptosis in cell cultures of human umbilical cord vascular endothelial cells (HUVEC) stressed with H_2O_2. Moreover, they increased the expression of the anti-apoptotic factor Bcl-2 in HUVECs. In an *in vivo* study the authors investigated injection of stressed EPC derived secretomes in a rodent model of hind limb ischaemia. This therapy increased hind limb blood flow, capillary density and improved muscle viability and functional performance. Additionally, injection of EPC secretomes induced the mobilization of bone marrow derived EPC and their homing to sites of ischaemia.

Based on these recent reports we sought to further investigate our hypothesis of cardioprotection induced by apoptotic cells particularly with regard to paracrine factors and their effects on cytoprotective, anti-apoptotic and regenerative processes.

Aims of the study

In the first part of the study, the mechanisms how apoptotic cells might modulate the remodelling process following AMI were investigated in a rodent model of LAD ligation. Based on our previous results [22], another way of cell administration, i.e. via intramyocardial injection was investigated. Moreover, a major goal of the study was to analyse the composition of the extracellular matrix of the myocardial scar tissue. Interestingly, a strong accumulation of elastic fibres was found in the cardiac scar tissue of animals injected with apoptotic cell suspensions. In order to further investigate this issue, RT-PCR analysis and immunohistology for growth factors inducing elastin expression was performed.

The goal of the second part of the study was to define signalling mechanisms how apoptotic cells can confer cardioprotective effects to the ischaemic myocardium. As paracrine effects were more and more in the focus of research on protection against myocardial ischaemia, cell culture supernatants of irradiated apoptotic PBMC were harvested, lyophilised in order to improve practicability (this compound was termed *APOSEC*, i.e. **apo**ptotic cell **sec**retome) and were injected in a rat model of AMI. Moreover, the mechanisms of cardioprotection mediated by apoptotic cell supernatants were investigated in various *in vitro* assays using human cardiac myocytes. As the administration of apoptotic cell derived supernatants showed convincing results in the small animal model and in *in vitro* assays, a porcine model of reperfused AMI was implemented. Using this type of animal model, it was possible to test the administration of apoptotic cell derived supernatants in an experimental setting that is much more comparable to the clinical scenario of AMI.

Materials and Methods

Descriptions of proceedings investigating the cardioprotective properties of apoptotic PBMC [34]

Acquisition of syngeneic rat PBMC suspensions for *in vivo* experiments

Experiments including animals were approved by the committee for animal research of the Medical University of Vienna and the Federal Ministry of Science and Research (ethics vote: BMBWK-66.009/0278-BrGT/2005). All animal experiments were performed in accordance to the Guide for the Care and Use of Laboratory Animals by the National Institutes of Health (NIH Publication No. 85-23). To obtain syngeneic rat PBMC for *in vivo* experiments, animals were anaesthetized and heparin was injected intravenously. Venous whole blood was aspirated by direct punctuation of the heart. Approximately 10-12 millilitres (ml) of blood were collected from each animal. The aspirated blood specimens were processed immediately and were diluted 1:2 in Hank's balanced salt solution HBSS (Lonza, Switzerland). The diluted blood suspensions were shifted carefully in a 50 ml tube containing Ficoll-Paque solution (GE Healthcare Bio-Sciences AB, Sweden). Tubes were centrifuged for 15 minutes at 800g at room temperature without brake. This cell separation technique generates a layer (buffy coat) of lymphocytes and monocytes in a very high degree of purity. Buffy coats of mononuclear cells were aspirated, washed once in HBSS and resuspended in 1 ml of fresh UltraCulture serum-free cell culture medium (Lonza, Switzerland). Cell concentrations were determined on a Sysmex automated cell counter (Sysmex Inc., USA).

    The separated PBMC suspensions were subjected to Caesium-137 irradiation (Department of Transfusion Medicine, General Hospital Vienna) with 45 Gray (Gy) in order to induce apoptotic cell death. Non-irradiated cells served as controls. The obtained cells were cultured in a humidified atmosphere for 18 hours. Induction of apoptosis was measured by using a co-staining for Annexin-V/Propidium iodine (Becton Dickinson, USA) on a flow cytometer. Annexin-positivity of PBMC was determined to be >80% and these cells were consequently classified as apoptotic PBMC (termed irradiated apoptotic PBMC, IA-PBMC).

Induction of acute myocardial infarction in male Sprague-Dawley rats

Acute myocardial infarction was induced in adult male Sprague-Dawley rats (weight 300 - 350g) by ligating the left anterior descending artery (LAD) as previously described [35, 36]. In short, animals were anaesthetized intraperitoneally with a mixture of xylazine (1mg per 100g bodyweight) and ketamine (10mg per 100g bodyweight), intubated using a venous catheter and ventilated mechanically. Rats were placed in a dorsal position and a left intercostal thoracotomy was performed and a ligature beneath the left atrium was placed around the LAD using 6-0 Prolene polypropylene suture. Immediately after the onset of ischaemia, cultured cell suspensions of $8.5*10^6$ viable or apoptotic PBMC suspended in 0.3 ml UltraCulture medium were injected into the femoral vein. In a second treatment group, apoptotic cells ($8.5 \cdot 10^6$ cells) were also injected directly into the myocardium at five different sites of the peri-infarct zone. Injection of cell culture medium alone and sham operation served as controls in this experimental setting. The mortality rate in these experiments was between 20% and 30%.

Histological and immunohistological evaluations

Tissue specimens were collected from animals that were sacrificed either 72 hours or 6 weeks after experimental infarction. A thoracotomy was performed, hearts were explanted and fixed in 10% neutral buffered formalin. Heart specimens were then sliced at three layers at the level of the largest extension of infarcted area (n=6 for 72 hours analyses, n=10-12 for 6 weeks analyses) and embedded in paraffin. The tissue samples were stained according to a haematoxylin-eosin (H&E) and Elastica van Gieson (EVG) staining protocol.

Immunohistological analysis of specimens obtained 72 hours after AMI was performed using antibodies directed to CD68 (MCA 341R, AbD Serotec, UK), c-kit (sc-168, Santa Cruz Biotechnology, USA), FLK1 (sc-6251, Santa Cruz Biotechnology, USA), IGF-I (sc-9013, Santa Cruz Biotechnology, USA) and FGF-2 (sc-79, Santa Cruz Biotechnology, USA). Specimens were evaluated on an Olympus AX70 microscope (Olympus Optical Co. Ltd., Japan) at a 200x magnification. Images were captured digitally using Meta Morph v4.5 Software (Molecular Devices, USA). Image J planimetry software (Rasband, W.S., Image J, U.S. National Institutes of Health, USA) was used to determine the area of necrosis after 72 hours and the dimension of myocardial infarction after 6 weeks. The extent of infarcted myocardial tissue (expressed as % of left ventricle) was calculated by dividing the area of the circumference of the infarcted area by the total endocardial and epicardial circumferenced areas of the left ventricle. Planimetric evaluation after six weeks was carried out on tissue samples stained with EVG for better comparison of vital myocardium and fibrotic areas. Infarction size was expressed as a percentage of the total left ventricular area. Tissue specimens stained with EVG were furthermore analysed microscopically for the ratio of elastic and collagen fibres within the left ventricular scar tissue. ImageJ planimetry software was utilized to calculate the elastin to collagen ratio by dividing the area occupied by elastic fibres by the total area of collagenous scar tissue.

Evaluation of cardiac function by echocardiography six weeks after induction of myocardial infarction

Animals were anaesthetized six weeks after induction of myocardial infarction as described above. Echocardiographic examination was conducted on a Vivid 7 system (General Electric Medical Systems, USA). All analyses were performed by an experienced observer blinded to the treatment groups to which the animals were allocated. M-mode tracings were recorded from a parasternal short-axis view and functional systolic and diastolic parameters were obtained (ejection fraction, EF; shortening fraction, SF; left ventricular end-diastolic diameter, LVEDD; left ventricular end-systolic diameter, LVESD, left ventricular end-diastolic volume, LVEDV; left ventricular end-systolic volume, LVESV). Ejection fraction was calculated as follows:

EF(%)=((LVEDV-LVESV)/LVEDV)*100. Shortening fractional was calculated as follows: SF(%)=((LVEDD – LVESD)/ LVEDD)*100.

Separation of human PBMC for *in vitro* experiments

Experimental procedures were approved by the local ethics committee of the Medical University of Vienna (ethics committee vote: EK-Nr 2010/034) and were conducted in compliance with the principles of the Declaration of Helsinki. Human peripheral blood mononuclear cells (PBMC) were obtained from young healthy volunteers by venous blood withdrawal after informed consent. Blood specimens in EDTA tubes were processed immediately and PBMC were obtained by Ficoll-Paque (GE Healthcare Bio-Sciences AB, Sweden) density gradient centrifugation as described above.

Apoptosis of PBMC was induced by Caesium-137 irradiation with 60 Gray (Gy) for *in vitro* experiments. Cells were resuspended in serum-free UltraCulture medium and cultured in a humidified atmosphere at 37° Celsius for 24 hours at a density of $2.5*10^6$ cells/ml, n=5). The induction of apoptosis in PBMC was measured by Annexin-V/Propidium iodine co-staining (Becton Dickinson, USA) on a flow cytometer. In order to characterize apoptotic cells, the Annexin-V-positivity of PBMC was determined to be >80%. Non-irradiated PBMC served as controls in all *in vitro* experiments and were termed "viable PBMC".

Moreover, supernatants of cell cultures of irradiated and non-irradiated cells were harvested after 24 hours and were stored at -80° Celsius until further analyses were conducted.

Cell culture of human fibroblasts exposed to supernatants of apoptotic PBMC, RNA isolation and cDNA preparation

Cell culture supernatants were obtained from viable PBMC, irradiated apoptotic PBMC and mixed co-cultures of viable and apoptotic cells after 24 hours (cell density $2.5*10^6$ resuspended in fresh UltraCulture medium) as described above. Human primary fibroblasts (Cascade Inc., USA), seeded at a density of $1*10^5$ cell per ml were exposed to supernatants obtained from viable PBMC, apoptotic PBMC and mixed cultures of viable and apoptotic cells for 24 hours. Fibroblasts were cultured in Dulbecco's modified Eagle medium (DMEM, Gibco BRL, USA) that was supplemented with 10% fetal bovine serum (FBS, PAA, Austria), 25mM L-glutamine (Gibco BRL, USA) and 1% penicillin/streptomycin (Gibco BRL, USA) and seeded in 12-well plates. After RNA extraction of fibroblasts (using RNeasy, QilAGEN, Austria) following the manufacturer's instruction, cDNAs were transcribed using the iScript cDNA synthesis kit (BioRad, USA).

Quantitative real time polymerase chain reaction (RT-PCR)

RT-PCR was used to quantify mRNA transcription of elastin, collagen type I, collagen type III, collagen type V, Interleukin 8 (IL-8), Matrixmetalloproteinase 1 (MMP1), Matrixmetalloproteinase 3 (MMP3) and Matrixmetalloproteinase 9 (MMP9). The expression of mRNA was quantified by RT-PCR on a LightCycler Fast Start DNA Master SYBR Green I (Roche Applied Science, Germany) according to the manufacturer's protocol. The primers for elastin (forward: 5´- CCTACTTACGGGGTTGG-3´, reverse: 5´- GCCGAGCAGACAAGAA-3´), collagen type I (forward: 5´- GTGCTAAAGGTGCCAATGGT-3´, reverse: 5´- CTCCTCGCTTTCCTTCCTCT-3´), collagen type III (forward: 5´- GTCCATGGATGGTGGTTTTC-3´, reverse: 5´- CACCTTCATTTGACCCCATC-3´), collagen type V (forward: 5´- GTCCATACCCGCTGGAAA-3´, reverse: 5´- TCCATCAGGCAAGTTGTGAA-3´), IL-8 (forward: 5´- CTCTTGGCAGCCTTCCTGATT-3´, reverse: 5´- TATGCACTGACATCTAAGTTCTTTAGCA-3´), MMP1 (forward: 5´- GGTCTCTGAGGGTCAAGCAG-3´, reverse: 5´- CCGCAACACGATGTAAGTTG-3´), MMP3 (forward: 5´- TGCTTTGTCCTTTGATGCTG-3´, reverse: 5´- GGCCCAGAATTGATTTCCTT-3´), MMP9 (forward: 5´- GGGAAGATGCTGGTGTTCA-3´, reverse: 5´-CCTGGCAGAAATAGGCTTC-3´) and β-2-microglobulin (β2M) (β2M, forward: 5´-GATGAGTATGCCTGCCGTGTG-3´, reverse: 5´-CAATCCAAATGCGGCATCT-3´) were designed as described previously

[37]. The relative expression of the target genes was calculated by comparison to the house keeping gene β2M using a formula as previously described [38].

Semi-quantitative evaluation of cytokines and growth factors secreted by apoptotic PBMC by means of membrane arrays

Cell culture supernatants of irradiated and non-irradiated human PBMC (cultured at a density of $2.5*10^6$/ml) were obtained from 4 healthy volunteers after informed consent. Membrane arrays for the detection of cytokines and growth factors in pooled supernatants were performed to analyse factors that are secreted by apoptotic cells in comparison to viable cells. Supernatants were screened for the presence and relative levels of a total of 274 cytokines by using a commercially available human cytokine antibody membrane array (AAH-CYT-4000, Ray Biotech, USA). Array experiments were performed according to the manufacturer's protocol. The obtained results were analysed using Image J software (Rasband, W.S., Image J, U.S. National Institutes of Health, USA). The secretion levels of each factor were expressed as relative to the respective positive controls in column 1 and 2 (VIABLE SN, APO SN). The fold increase over non-irradiated cell culture supernatants was expressed in column 3 (APO SN divided by VIABLE SN), see Table 1.

Descriptions of proceedings investigating the cardioprotective properties of cell culture supernatants of apoptotic PBMC (APOSEC) [39]

Production of APOSEC^H, APOSEC^R and APOSEC^P – Supernatants derived from irradiated apoptotic PBMC

Human peripheral blood mononuclear cells (PBMC) were obtained from young healthy volunteers after informed consent as described above. Apoptosis of PBMC was induced by Caesium-137 irradiation with 60 Gray. Irradiated and non-irradiated cells were resuspended in fresh serum-free UltraCulture Medium (Lonza, Switzerland) and cultured for 24 hours in various cell densities ($1 \cdot 10^6$, $2.5 \cdot 10^6$ and $25 \cdot 10^6$ cells/ml, n=5) in a humidified atmosphere at 37° Celsius. After 24 hours, supernatants were collected and were subjected to ELISA content analysis or were lyophilised for further experiments. For lyophilisation, cell culture supernatants were dialyzed against ammonium acetate (at a concentration of 50mM) over night at 4°C. The obtained liquid (APOSEC^H) was sterile filtered using a 0.2µm filter (Whatman Filter 0.2µm FP30/o,2 Ca-S, Germany), frozen and lyophilised overnight (Lyophilisator Christ alpha 1-4, Martin Christ Gefriertrocknungsanlagen GmbH, Germany).

For *in vivo* rat experiments, syngeneic rat PBMC were separated by density gradient centrifugation from venous whole blood obtained from heparinized rats as described above. PBMC were irradiated by Caesium-137 (45 Gy) and cultured for 24 hours at a cell density of $25 \cdot 10^6$ cells/ml (resuspended in UltraCulture medium, Lonza, Switzerland). APOSEC for *in vivo* rat experiments (APOSEC^R) was further processed as described for APOSEC^H. Supernatants of non-irradiated rat PBMC cell cultures and fresh UltraCulture medium served as controls.

For large animal experiments, blood was obtained from anaesthetized pigs by direct puncture of the heart. Three pigs were anaesthetized with an intravenous bolus injection of 10 mg/kg ketamine and 1.3 mg/kg azaperone. A left thoracic dermal incision was conducted and a direct puncture of the heart was then performed under sterile conditions using a hollow needle. Arterial blood was drawn using 50 ml syringes. Blood obtained in syringes during this procedure was immediately transferred into heparinised plastic bags (3000 ml) for blood products. PBMC were then obtained according to the same protocol as described above. CellGro serum-free medium (Cell Genix, Germany), a *"Good Manufacturing Practice"* certified culture medium, was utilized for porcine PBMC derived APOSEC production (APOSEC^P). APOSEC for porcine experiments (APOSEC^P) was processed as described for APOSEC^H.

In order to avoid possible cross-species detrimental immune reactions, we opted to utilize APOSEC preparations solely in a syngeneic fashion (human APOSEC, APOSEC^H; rat APOSEC, APOSEC^R; porcine APOSEC, APOSEC^P).

Membrane array and ELISA analysis of cytokines and growth factors in APOSEC^H

Human PBMC derived APOSEC (APOSEC^H) was screened for cytokines and angiogenic factors using two commercially available array systems (ARY005, ARY007, Proteome Profiler Arrays, R&D Systems, USA). Membrane array experiments were performed according the manufacturer's instructions. Moreover, supernatant levels of cytokines and growth factors secreted by irradiated and non-irradiated PBMC in various concentrations ($1·10^6$, $2.5·10^6$ and $25·10^6$ cells/ml, n=5) were measured by utilizing commercially available enzyme-linked immunosorbent assay systems (ELISA, Duoset, R&D Systems, USA) kits for the quantification of IL-8, GRO-α, ENA-78, VEGF, IL-16, IL-10, TGF-β, sICAM-1, RANTES, IL-1ra, MIF, PAI-1, IGF-I, HGF, FGF-2, MCP-1, MMP9, SDF-1, G-CSF, GM-CSF and HMGB1 (IBL International GmbH, Germany). In brief, ninety-six–well plates (Nunc Maxisorp plates, Nunc GmbH & Co. KG, Germany) were coated overnight with capture antibodies at room temperature. After blocking of plates, supernatant samples and standard proteins were added to the wells. After a two hour incubation period and a washing step, a biotin-labelled antibody was added to each well and incubated for an additional two hours. Plates were washed and streptavidin-horseradish peroxidase was added. Colour reaction was achieved using a tetramethylbenzidine substrate solution (TMB; Sigma Aldrich, USA) and was stopped by a 1N sulphuric acid stop solution (Merck, Germany). Immediately thereafter, optical density values were measured at 450 nm on a plate reader (Victor3 Multilabel plate reader, PerkinElmer, USA).

Rat AMI model and APOSEC^R treatment

Small animal experiments investigating APOSEC^R administration in rats were approved by the committee for animal research, Medical University of Vienna and the Federal Ministry of Science and Research (vote: 66.009/0168-II/10b/2008). Acute myocardial infarction was induced in adult male Sprague-Dawley rats (weight 275-300g) by ligating the LAD as described previously. Immediately after the onset of myocardial ischaemia, lyophilised supernatants obtained from $8.5 \cdot 10^6$ either irradiated apoptotic PBMC or non-irradiated viable cells resuspended in 0.3 ml fresh UltraCulture medium (Lonza, Switzerland) were injected into the femoral vein. The administration of fresh UltraCulture cell culture medium served as negative control. In sham operated animals a left lateral thoracotomy was performed but no ligation was placed around the LAD.

Histological and immunohistological analysis and determination of myocardial infarction size by planimetry

Rats were sacrificed either 72 hours or 6 weeks after experimental infarction was induced. Hearts were explanted, placed in formalin overnight and were then sliced in three layers at the level of the largest extension of infarcted area (n=6 for 72 hours analyses, n=9 for 6 weeks analyses). The obtained tissue samples were stained according to a haematoxylin-eosin (H&E) and Elastica van Gieson (EVG) protocol. Short-term immunohistological evaluation on specimens obtained 72 hours after induction of AMI was performed using antibodies directed to CD68 (MCA341R, AbD Serotec, UK) and c-kit (sc-168, Santa Cruz Biotechnology, USA). Image J planimetry software (Rasband, W.S., Image J, U.S. National Institutes of Health, USA) was utilized in order to measure the extent of myocardial infarction after 6 weeks.

Enzymatic digestion of infarcted myocardium and flow cytometric analysis

Hearts were explanted from 6 rats with LAD ligation three days after infarction was induced (n=3 APOSEC injected rats, n=3 medium controls). The infarcted areas of explanted hearts were excised, cut into small cubic pieces (1mm in diameter) and incubated with collagenase (2.4 U/ml, Sigma Aldrich, USA) for 12 hours at 4°C as previously described [40, 41]. After that digestion period, cell suspensions were washed and obtained cells were subsequently incubated with primary antibodies directed to CD68 (MCA341R, AbD Serotec, UK) and c-kit (sc-168, Santa Cruz Biotechnology, USA). After an incubation period with a secondary antibody, cell suspensions were analysed for total CD68+ and c-kit+ cell numbers by means of flow cytometry (FACS Calibur, Becton Dickinson, USA).

Assessment of cardiac function by means of echocardiography

Echocardiographic examinations were conducted on a Vivid 7 system (General Electric Medical Systems, USA) as previously described. All measurements were performed by an experienced evaluator blinded to treatment or control groups. Values for left ventricular ejection fraction (EF), shortening fraction (SF), left ventricular end-systolic diameters (LVESD), left ventricular end-diastolic diameters (LVEDD), left ventricular end-systolic volumes (LVESV) and left ventricular end-diastolic volumes (LVEDV) were assessed.

Large animal AMI model

In order to investigate the cardioprotective effects of APOSEC preparations, we opted for a large animal model of the clinically more relevant setting of ischaemia and reperfusion. For this setting, the porcine closed chest reperfused AMI infarction model was chosen [42-44]. In this model, conditions are more similar to those in human AMI and primary percutaneous coronary intervention (PCI) than in any other animal model, and they thus allow a translational research approach. These large animal experiments were conducted at the Institute of Diagnostics and Oncoradiology, University of Kaposvar, Hungary and were approved by the University of Kaposvar (ethics vote: 246/002/SOM2006, MAB-28-2005).

In total, 32 adolescent pigs (female Large Whites weighing approximately 30kg) were sedated with 12 mg/kg ketamine hydrochloride, 1 mg/kg xylazine and 0.04 mg/kg atropine. An intratracheal intubation was then performed to maintain thorough anaesthesia with a mixture of isoflurane, O_2 and N_2O. During anaesthesia, O_2 saturation and electrocardiography were monitored continuously. Vascular access to the right femoral artery and the right femoral vein was performed and 6 Fr (French scale) and 7 Fr introduction sheaths were then inserted into artery and vein, respectively. Heparin (200 IU/kg) was administered and a 6 Fr guiding catheter (Medtronic Inc., USA) was introduced into the left coronary ostium and a coronary angiography was performed (using Ultravist contrast medium, Bayer Healthcare, Germany).

For the induction of AMI, a balloon catheter (diameter: 3 mm, length: 15 mm; Boston Scientific, USA) was inserted into the LAD right after the origin of the second major diagonal branch. The LAD was then subsequently occluded by inflating the balloon slowly at 4 – 6 standard atmospheres (atm), (n=11 animals in the control group, n=10 in the treatment high dose and n=7 in the treatment low dose group). The occlusion of the LAD was controlled with angiography. Forty minutes after start of the occlusion, the lyophilised supernatant obtained from $250 \cdot 10^6$ (low dose group), $1 \cdot 10^9$ (high dose group) irradiated apoptotic porcine PBMC or lyophilised serum-free cell culture medium (CellGro Medium, Cell Genix, Germany) was resuspended in 250 ml of 0.9% physiologic sodium chloride solution and was administered intravenously over the next 25 minutes. 90 minutes after LAD occlusion, the balloon was slowly deflated and reperfusion was established again. A control coronary angiography was performed to prove the patency of the infarct-related artery and to exclude arterial injury in all animals. Moreover, all animals received 75mg clopidogrel and 100mg acetylsalicylic acid.

In situ viability staining using tetrazolium chloride

Either 24 hours or 30 days after AMI, euthanasia was performed by the administration of saturated potassium chloride. In order to delineate infarcted (necrotic) areas and areas at risk for ischaemia *in situ* double-staining with 1% Evans blue dye and a 4% solution of 2,3,5-triphenyltetrazolium chloride (TTC) was performed after 24 hours. In short, after explantation of the heart, the LAD was occluded again at same position where the balloon was situated before and both coronary arteries were perfused with an Evans blue solution to delineate the area at risk and non-risk regions of the myocardium. The hearts were cut in into 7 mm thick slices starting from the apex towards the level of the occlusion (6-7 layers per heart). The slices were then incubated in 500 ml of TTC solution at 37 °C in a shaking water bath for 20 minutes. Subsequently, all slices underwent an overnight bleach cycle at room temperature in 4,5% formalin. After bleaching, slices were photographed using a digital camera (Panasonic HDC-HS700, Japan) mounted on a fixed stand. Planimetric analysis was performed using Image J software (Rasband, W.S., Image J, U.S. National Institutes of Health, USA).

Hearts of all animals in the 30 days follow-up groups were fixed in formalin and embedded in paraffin for histological staining (H&E, Movat's pentachrome staining).

In order to prove that the coronary circulation was comparable between all three treatment groups, the Bypass Angioplasty Revascularization Investigation Myocardial Jeopardy Index (BARI score) was calculated based on LAD and LCX pre-occlusion angiograms as previously described [45].

Measurement of Troponin I levels after AMI

Serum samples were obtained from venous blood at the start of the experimental procedure, at the start of reperfusion and after 24 hours. Levels of Troponin I were determined by ELISA (Uscn Life Science Inc., China) according to the manufacturer's instructions.

Determination of cardiac functional parameters after AMI by magnetic resonance imaging (MRI)

Cardiac MRI was performed using a 1.5-T clinical scanner (Avanto, Siemens, Germany) three and 30 days after LAD occlusion as previously described [46]. MR images were acquired using a retrospectively ECG-gated, steady-state free precession cine MRI technique in short-axis and long-axis views of the heart. Delayed enhancement images were obtained after injection of 0.05 mmol/kg of contrast medium, short-axis and long-axis images were obtained 10 to 15 minutes after injection. The images were analysed using Mass 6.1.6 software (Medis, The Netherlands). After segmentation of the left ventricular endocardial and epicardial borders, end-diastolic and end-systolic volumes and left ventricular ejection fractions were calculated. The left ventricular and infarcted myocardial mass was determined from the cine and delayed enhancement MR images. The extent of myocardial infarction was expressed relative to the left ventricular mass. Data analyses and interpretations were performed by an experienced observer blinded to all study results.

Cell culture of primary human cardiomyocytes and immunoblot analysis

Primary human ventricular cardiac myocytes were obtained (CellSystems Biotechnologie, Germany) and cultured in cardiac myocyte medium (CellSystems Biotechnologie, Germany) at 37°C. In order to investigate the cytoprotective activity of APOSEC preparations, $3 \cdot 10^5$ human cardiomyocytes were seeded in 6-well plates and cultivated in either basal medium without serum and growth factors or in basal medium supplemented with APOSEC^H (APOSEC derived from $0.25 \cdot 10^6$, $2.5 \cdot 10^6$ and $25 \cdot 10^6$ PBMC) for 24 hours.

For Western Blot analysis, $3 \cdot 10^5$ human cardiac myocytes were incubated with APOSEC^H (PBMC cell density for APOSEC production, $2.5 \cdot 10^6$ per ml) or with lyophilised UltraCulture medium for 5, 10, 30 and 60 minutes and for 24 hours. Immunodetection was performed with anti-phospho-c-Jun (1 µg/ml, New England Biolabs, USA), anti-phospho-CREB (1 µg/ml, New England Biolabs, USA), anti-phospho-AKT (1 µg/ml, New England Biolabs, USA), anti-phospho-Erk1/2 (1 µg/ml, New England Biolabs, USA), anti-phospho-Hsp27 (Ser15) (1 µg/ml, New England Biolabs, USA), anti-phospho-Hsp27 (Ser85), anti-phospho-BAG1 (C-16) (1 µg/ml, Santa Cruz Biotechnology, Germany), anti-Bcl-2 (2µg/ml, Acris, Germany), followed by horseradish peroxidase-conjugated goat anti-rabbit or goat anti-mouse IgG antisera (dilution 1:10000; Amersham BioSciences, Germany). In parallel, identical blots were performed for the equivalent non-phosporylated factors as controls. Moreover, a membrane-array (R&D Systems) analysing apoptosis mediating factors was performed with lysates from cardiac myocytes treated with either medium or APOSEC^H (PBMC cell density $2.5 \cdot 10^6$) for 24 hours according to the manufacturer's instructions.

Statistical methods

All statistical analyses were performed using Graph Pad Prism software (Graph Pad Software, USA). Data are shown as mean ± standard error of the mean (SEM). The Wilcoxon-Mann-Whitney-test or Student's t-test were utilized to calculate significances between groups. In boxplot figures, whiskers indicate minimums and maximums, the upper edge of the box indicates the 75th percentile and the lower one indicates the 25th percentile. P-values <0.05 were considered statistically significant.

Results

Results of experiments investigating the cardioprotective properties of apoptotic PBMC [34]

Histological analysis of cardiac specimens obtained three days after AMI

Three days after ligation of the LAD, hearts were explanted, fixed in formalin and stained histologically by means of H&E histology. In control animals and rats injected with non-irradiated viable PBMC, the cellular infiltrate in the infarcted myocardium evidenced a mixed pattern consisting of neutrophils, monocytes /macrophages and dystrophic or necrotic cardiac myocytes. In both treatment groups (intravienious injection of IA-PBMC, intramyocardial injection of IA-PBMC), the cellular infiltrate appeared more monomorphic and much denser compared to controls.

An analysis of cardiac sections performed three days after AMI by means of planimetry evidenced a significant reduction of the total infarcted area.

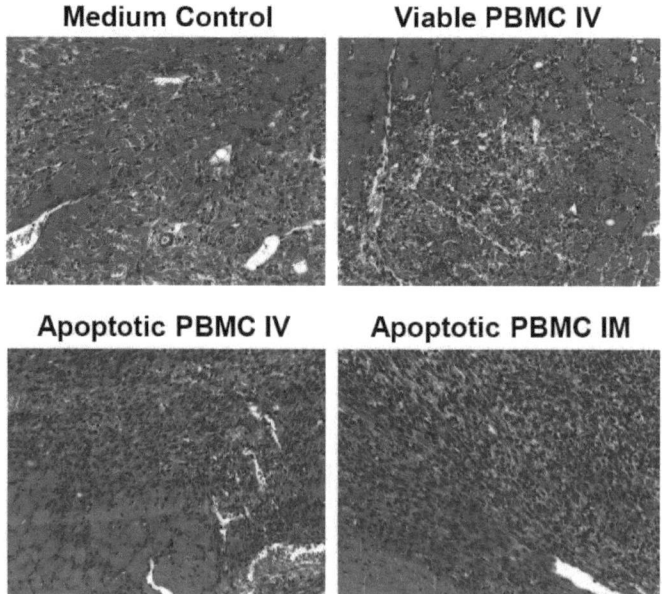

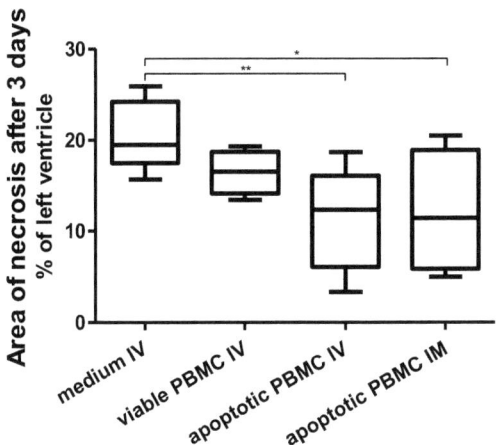

Figure 5 shows representative images of H&E stained specimens obtained three days after infarction and a quantification of the infarcted myocardium by planimetry.

Immunohistological staining for CD68, c-kit and VEGF receptor 2

In order to further characterize the cellular infiltrate we performed analyses by immunohistology for the markers CD68 (expressed on macrophages) and c-kit and VEGF receptor 2 (FLK1), both expressed on endothelial progenitor cells (EPC). Compared to the two control groups, much higher numbers of cells staining positive for CD68 were found in rats injected with irradiated apoptotic PBMC. The highest numbers were detected in animals that underwent direct intramyocardial injection of IA-PBMC. Moreover, the number of cells staining positive for the markers c-kit and FLK1 was increased in rats that were injected with IA-PBMC (either intravenously or intramyocardially), especially in the epicardial regions of the infarcted myocardium.

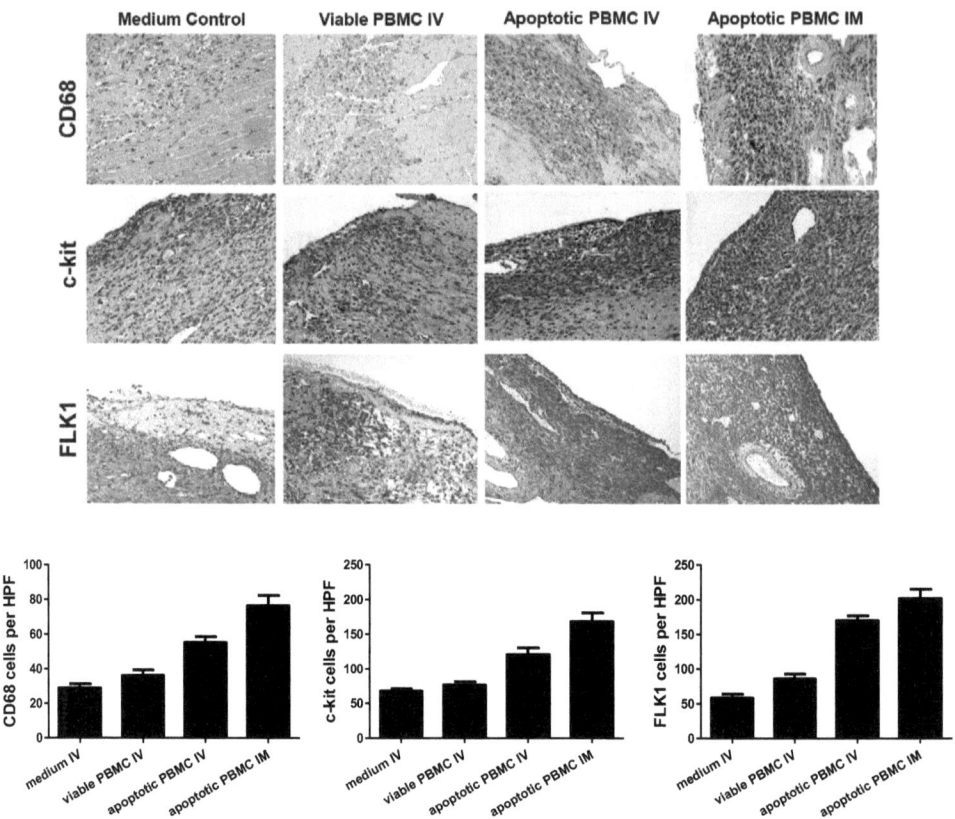

Figure 6 shows representative images of heart specimens stained for CD68, c-kit and FLK1 by means of immunohistology. Bar charts show the results obtained by quantification of high power fields (HPF).

The total number of cells quantified per high power-field (HPF) were 28.6±2.4 (±SEM) in control animals, 36.0±3.5 (±SEM) in animals injected with non-irradiated viable cells compared to 55.3±3.4 and 76.5±5.9 (±SEM) in rats injected with irradiated apoptotic cells (IV or IM, respectively). Within the infiltrate, most of the monocytic cells were identified to be highly positive for the marker c-kit and FLK1. HPF cell counts for c-kit were 68.0±3.1 (±SEM) in controls, 77.0±4.6 (±SEM) in rats that were injected with viable cell compared to 121.2±9.4 (±SEM) in intravenously (IV) and 168.6±12.4 (±SEM) in intramyocardially (IM) injected animals (see Figure 6). In specimens stained for FLK-1, these values were 58.3±5.6 (±SEM) in controls,

86.0±7.0 (±SEM) for viable cell injected rats, 170.3±7.1 (±SEM) for intravenously and 202.0±9.4 (±SEM) for intramyocardially injected animals (see Figure 6, n=5-6 per group).

Histological evaluation six weeks after LAD ligation

In order to determine the extent of fibrotic scar tissue within the left ventricular myocardium, cardiac specimens obtained six weeks after induction of AMI by LAD ligation were stained with Elastica van Gieson staining. A significant reduction in regards to scar dimension was found for animals injected with suspension of irradiated PBMC compared to controls. In both control groups, large infarct were common (between 14% and 25% of the left ventricle) whereas a significant reduction to values between 6% and 8% was evident in rats treated with apoptotic PBMC ($p<0.01$ vs. controls, $p<0.05$ vs. viable cell injected animals, n=10-12 per group). Moreover, the ventricular geometry was almost completely preserved in treated animals whereas signs of dilation could be found in animals injected with medium or non-irradiated cells.

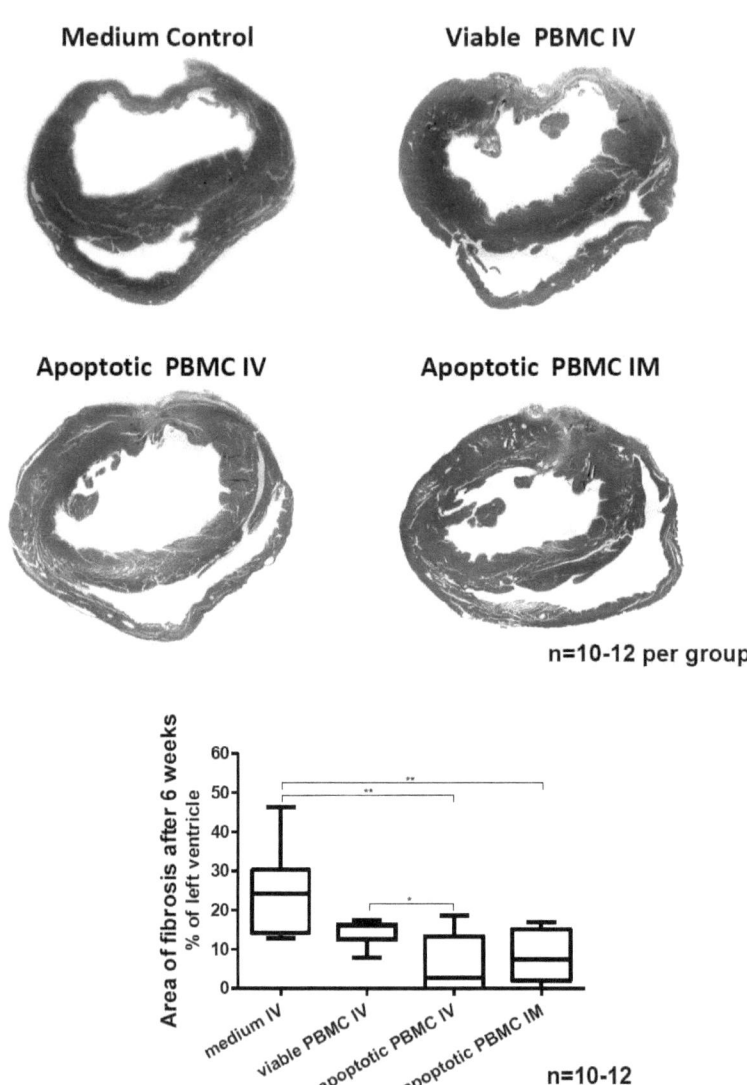

Figure 7 Hearts explanted from apoptotic cell injected rats six weeks after induction of AMI evidenced less myocardial damage compared to controls. Hearts obtained from medium as well as from viable cell injected rats appear more dilated and furthermore also show a greater extension of fibrotic tissue. A planimetric analysis performed on specimens collected six weeks after LAD ligation showed a mean scar extension of 25% in medium injected controls, 14% in viable cell injected animals compared to 6% (IV) and 8% (IM) in rats adminstered with apoptotic PBMC.

Assessment of cardiac function by echocardiography

Six weeks after induction of AMI by LAD ligation, all animals were sedated and parameters of cardiac function were assessed by means of echocardiography. In healthy rats without induction of AMI (i.e. sham operated animals) functional parameters were as follows: 60% ±4 (left ventricular ejection, EF), 29% ±2 (shortening fraction, SF), 9.2mm ±0.4 (left ventricular end-diastolic diameter, LVEDD), 6.5 mm ±0.3 (left ventricular end-systolic diameter, LVESD), 1.7 ml ±0.3 (left ventricular end-diastolic volume, LVEDV) and 0.7 ml ±0.1 (left ventricular end-systolic volume, LVESV). In control animals (injection of culture medium) mean EF, SF, LVEDD, LVESD, LVEDV and LVESV were impaired: 43% ±2 (EF), 19% ±1 (SF), 10.4 mm ±0.2 (LVEDD), 8.5 mm ±0.2 (LVESD), 2.3 ml ±0.1 (LVEDV) and 1.3 ml ±0.1 (LVESV). This was also true for animals that were injected with non-irradiated viable PBMC suspensions as evidenced by similar values: 42% ±3 (EF), 18% ±2 (SF), 11.0 mm ±0.4 (LVEDD), 9.0 mm ±0.5 (LVESD), 2.7 ml ±0.3 (LVEDV) and 1.6 ml ±0.2 (LVESV).

A significant improvement of regards to functional parameters were found in rats with intravenous injection of apoptotic cell suspensions: 53% ±4 (EF), 25% ±3 (SF), 8.9 mm ±0.3 (LVEDD), 6.8 mm ±0.4 (LVESD), 1.6 ml ±0.2 (LVEDV) and 0.8 ml ±0.1 (LVESV). Concomitantly, animals that underwent direct intramyocardial injection of apoptotic cell suspensions, these functional parameters were improved as well: 55% ±4 (EF), 26% ±2 (SF), 9.8 mm ±0.4 (LVEDD), 7.4 mm ±0.5 (LVESD), 2.1 ml ±0.2 (LVEDV) and 0.9 ml ±0.2 (LVESV).

Analysis of the composition of left ventricular scar tissue six weeks after AMI

By analysing Elastica van Gieson stained cardiac specimens obtained six weeks after AMI the composition of the fibrotic scar tissue was evaluated microscopically. Of special interest was the border zone between viable myocardium and scar tissue where a highly remarkably accumulation of elastic fibres was detected in animals injected with apoptotic cells in comparison to controls. To a lesser extent this phenomenon was also detectable in rats injected with viable cell suspensions. By utilizing planimetry software, it was shown that the fibrotic scar in apoptotic cell (IV and IM) injected rats was composed by 5.5%±1.1 and 8.9%±2.2 of elastic fibres compared to 0.2%±0.1 in controls and 2.9%±0.2 in viable injected animals, (p<0.001 vs. control, n=10-12 animals per group).

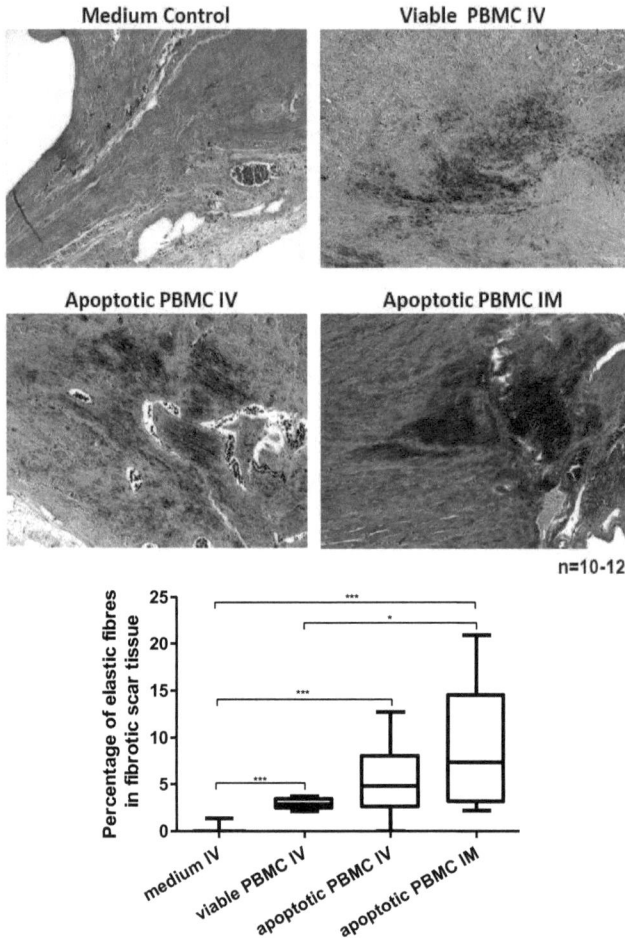

Figure 8: shows the accumulation of elastic fibres in the border zone between viable myocardium and scar tissue. Injection of apoptotic cells significantly increased elastin accumulation.

These higher amounts of elastic fibre accumulation stands in relation to higher levels of cells staining positively for Insulin-like growth factor I (IGF-I) and Fibroblast growth factor 2 (FGF-2) in treated animals compared to controls: rats injected with apoptotic

PBMC suspensions evidenced 36.0±3.3 cells staining positively for IGF-I per high power field (HPF) and 49.8±5.2 for FGF-2 per HPF in immunohistological analyses of cardiac specimens obtained 72 hours after induction of AMI. In comparison, only 7.0±1.6 IGF-I and 31.5±2.3 FGF-2 positive cells were detectable in control animals.

In order to further specify the association of elastin and collagen production within myocardial scar tissue and mechanisms induced by apoptotic cells, RT-PCR analyses were conducted. When exposing fibroblasts to cell culture supernatants obtained from apoptotic PBMC or apoptotic cells co-incubated with viable cells, elastin expression increased only slightly by 1.2 to 1.4 fold. The expression of collagen type III and IV increased moderately by 1.9 to 2.5 fold compared to controls (Fig. 3I). Supernatants derived from apoptotic cells also increased the expression of IL-8 (4-6.5 fold), MMP1 (18-31 fold), MMP3 (10-16 fold) and MMP9 (4-7 fold) in fibroblasts indicating a mechanistic cross-talk between apoptotic cells, their secretome and resident cells that could be accounted for alterations in the compositions of the extracellular matrix.

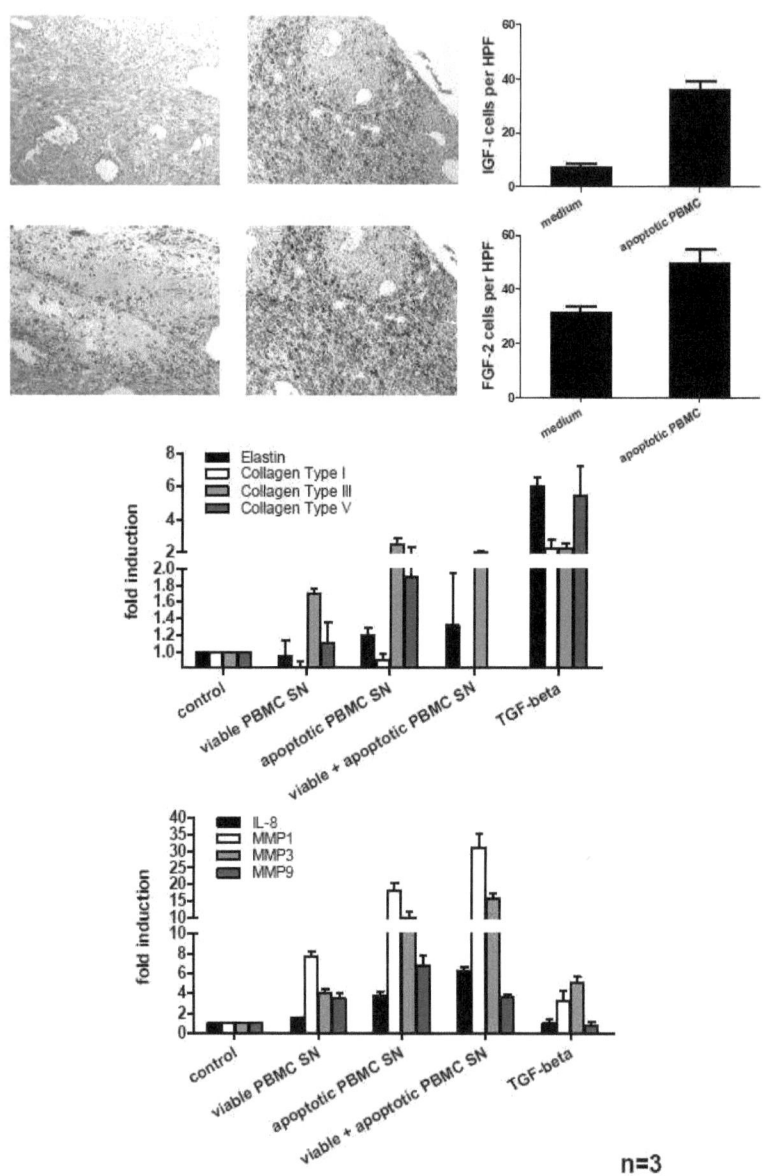

Figure 9 show immunohistological tissue sections stained for IGF-I and FGF-2 in controls and treated animals. Below data from RT-PCR analyses is shown. Human fibroblasts incubated with supernatants (SN) derived from apoptotic cells increased expression of elastin, collagen type III and IV, IL-8, MMP1, MMP3 and MMP9 transcripts.

Different secretion patterns of cytokines, chemokines and growth factors in apoptotic cells

Based on the finding in RT-PCR analysis that the expression of transcripts for IL-8 and MMPs was up-regulated in apoptotic PBMC, culture supernatants obtained from irradiated apoptotic and non-irradiated viable cells were analysed for 274 cytokines and growth factors by membrane arrays. Considerable differences were observed (amongst others) for IL-8, VEGF, MMP3, MMP9, IL-16, ENA-78 and MIP-1alpha (see table below). The results were analysed using Image J software. The secretion levels were expressed as relative to the respective positive control in column 1 and 2 (VIABLE SN, APO SN). The fold increase over supernatants obtained from non-irradiated cells was expressed in column 3 (APO SN divided by VIABLE SN).

Cytokines	VIABLE SN	APO SN	Fold increase	Cytokines	VIABLE SN	APO SN	Fold increase
Eotaxin-2	0,08	0,01	0,07	CTACK	0,02	0,04	1,79
IGF-I	0,07	0,06	0,90	ICAM-1	0,25	0,47	1,86
Leptin	0,06	0,06	1,02	I-TAC	not detect.	not detect.	not detect.
PDGF-BB	0,92	0,67	0,73	TECK	not detect.	not detect.	not detect.
Eotaxin-3	not detect.	not detect.	not detect.	Dtk	not detect.	not detect.	not detect.
IL-10	not detect.	not detect.	not detect.	ICAM-3	not detect.	not detect.	not detect.
LIGHT	not detect.	not detect.	not detect.	Lymphotactin	0,05	0,07	1,41
RANTES	0,97	1,74	1,80	TIMP-1	0,30	0,44	1,46
FGF-6	0,07	0,06	0,81	EGF-R	0,08	0,03	0,45
IL-13	not detect.	not detect.	not detect.	IGFBP-3	0,13	0,15	1,16
MCP-1	0,23	0,23	0,99	MIF	0,19	0,43	2,24
SCF	not detect.	not detect.	not detect.	TIMP-2	0,26	0,45	1,72
FGF-7	not detect.	0,06	APO SN only	ENA-78	0,21	0,56	2,66
IL-15	not detect.	not detect.	not detect.	IGFBP-6	0,14	0,35	2,43
MCP-2	0,15	0,07	0,48	MIP-1α	0,05	0,13	2,45
SDF-1	not detect.	not detect.	not detect.	Thrombopoietin	0,02	0,06	2,43
Flt-3 Ligand	not detect.	not detect.	not detect.	Fas/TNFRSF6	0,18	0,33	1,85
IL-16	0,15	0,75	4,99	IGF-I SR	0,03	0,05	1,89
MCP-3	0,07	0,09	1,19	MIP-1β	0,16	0,16	0,97
TARC	0,13	not detect.	VIABLE SN only	TRAIL R3	0,15	0,36	2,40
Angiogenin	0,67	0,92	1,37	Acrp30	1,22	2,19	1,80
Fractalkine	not detect.	not detect.	not detect.	FGF-4	0,21	0,34	1,61
IL-1α	0,09	0,02	0,27	IL-1 R4/ST2	0,05	0,04	0,87
MCP-4	not detect.	not detect.	not detect.	MIP-3β	not detect.	not detect.	not detect.
TGF-β1	0,11	0,05	0,48	TRAIL R4	not detect.	not detect.	not detect.
BDNF	0,42	0,44	1,05	AgRP	0,07	0,09	1,39

GCP-2	not detect.	not detect.	not detect.	FGF-9	0,18	0,22	1,24
IL-1β	0,17	0,06	0,36	IL-1 RI	0,06	0,19	2,99
M-CSF	0,11	0,11	1,00	MSP-α	0,27	0,45	1,67
TGF-β 3	not detect.	0,08	APO SN only	uPAR	0,27	0,41	1,48
BLC	not detect.	not detect.	not detect.	Angiopoietin-2	0,15	0,30	1,98
GDNF	not detect.	not detect.	not detect.	GCSF	not detect.	not detect.	not detect.
IL-1ra	0,27	0,43	1,62	IL-11	not detect.	not detect.	not detect.
MDC	0,16	0,29	1,83	NT-4	0,08	0,09	1,08
TNF-α	0,10	0,05	0,53	VEGF	0,08	0,25	3,34
BMP-4	0,16	0,20	1,28	Amphiregulin	0,10	0,13	1,40
GM-CSF	not detect.	not detect.	not detect.	GITR-Ligand	0,08	0,12	1,58
IL-2	not detect.	not detect.	not detect.	IL-12 p40	0,22	0,55	2,49
MIG	not detect.	not detect.	not detect.	Osteoprotegerin	0,06	0,10	1,82
TNF-β	0,14	0,13	0,92	VEGF-D	0,08	0,23	2,86
BMP-6	0,14	not detect.	VIABLE SN only	Axl	0,13	0,13	0,96
I-309	0,27	0,25	0,91	GITR	0,13	0,16	1,22
IL-3	0,24	0,24	0,99	IL-12 p70	0,08	0,11	1,42
MIP-1δ	0,15	0,11	0,71	Oncostatin M	0,11	0,19	1,78
CK β 8-1	0,15	0,16	1,09	bFGF	0,03	0,06	1,95
IFN-γ	not detect.	not detect.	not detect.	GRO	0,65	1,06	1,63
IL-4	not detect.	not detect.	not detect.	IL-17	not detect.	not detect.	not detect.
MIP-3α	0,25	0,16	0,64	PIGF	0,15	0,24	1,61
CNTF	not detect.	not detect.	not detect.	b-NGF	0,03	0,05	1,61
IGFBP-1	not detect.	not detect.	not detect.	GRO-α	0,25	0,33	1,36
IL-5	not detect.	not detect.	not detect.	IL-2 R alpha	0,09	0,22	2,54
NAP-2	0,48	0,77	1,61	sgp130	0,15	0,29	1,94
EGF	0,74	1,00	1,34	BTC	0,11	0,13	1,23
IGFBP-2	0,10	0,10	1,08	HCC-4	0,07	0,11	1,47
IL-6	0,34	0,05	0,15	IL-6 R	0,34	0,85	2,47
NT-3	0,16	0,18	1,13	sTNF RII	0,35	0,77	2,20
Eotaxin	not detect.	not detect.	not detect.	CCL-28	not detect.	not detect.	not detect.
IGFBP-4	0,10	0,20	2,05	HGF	0,18	0,16	0,89
IL-7	not detect.	not detect.	not detect.	IL-8	0,43	1,48	3,44
PARC	not detect.	not detect.	not detect.	sTNF-RI	0,12	0,12	0,99
Endoglin	not detect.	not detect.	not detect.	Furin	0,12	0,13	1,10
IL-21R	not detect.	not detect.	not detect.	LYVE-1	0,15	0,17	1,09
PDGF AA	0,34	0,40	1,18	Osteopontin	0,10	0,07	0,71
VE-Cadherin	not detect.	not detect.	not detect.	Trappin-2	0,05	0,09	1,87
ErbB3	0,08	0,07	0,92	Galectin-7	not detect.	not detect.	not detect.
IL-5 R alpha	0,04	0,07	1,74	Marapsin	0,07	0,06	0,84
PDGF-AB	0,18	0,20	1,06	PAI-I	0,19	0,30	1,60
VEGF R2	0,06	not detect.	VIABLE SN only	TREM-1	0,05	0,06	1,29
E-Selectin	0,09	0,12	1,25	GDF-15	0,13	0,13	1,03
IL-9	0,11	0,11	0,99	MICA	0,07	0,07	0,97
PDGF-R alpha	not detect.	not detect.	not detect.	Platelet Factor 4	0,11	0,14	1,23
VEGF R3	0,18	0,20	1,06	TSH	0,05	0,06	1,40

Fas Ligand	0,13	0,07	0,57	Growth Hormon	0,05	0,04	0,78
IP-10	0,14	0,16	1,16	MICB	0,09	0,08	0,92
PDGF-R beta	not detect.	not detect.	not detect.	PSA-total	0,07	0,08	1,15
ICAM-2	0,28	0,46	1,66	TSLP	not detect.	not detect.	not detect.
LAP	0,24	0,33	1,38	Adiposin	0,29	0,43	1,49
PECAM-1	0,11	0,10	0,96	IL-10 R alpha	0,09	0,15	1,64
Activin A	not detect.	not detect.	not detect.	MMP-2	0,08	0,12	1,47
IGF-II	0,17	0,22	1,29	RAGE	0,05	0,10	2,07
Leptin R	0,05	0,07	1,37	VCAM-1	0,05	0,07	1,35
Prolactin	0,09	0,07	0,86	BCAM	0,09	0,12	1,39
ALCAM	0,17	0,22	1,30	IL-22	0,07	0,09	1,35
IL-1 R II	0,06	0,05	0,77	MMP-7	0,12	0,13	1,10
LIF	0,14	0,15	1,09	RANK	0,09	0,07	0,88
SCF R	0,27	0,28	1,04	VEGF-C	0,15	0,14	0,91
B7-1(CD80)	0,14	0,08	0,58	CD30	0,12	0,16	1,27
IL-10 R beta	not detect.	not detect.	not detect.	IL-28A	0,19	0,21	1,12
L-Selectin	0,21	0,23	1,07	MMP-8	0,19	0,30	1,54
SDF-1beta	not detect.	not detect.	not detect.	Resistin	0,08	0,08	0,97
BMP-5	0,24	0,17	0,73	XEDAR	0,07	0,10	1,39
IL-13 R alpha 2	0,17	0,25	1,46	CD40	0,06	0,05	0,89
M-CSF R	0,20	0,40	1,99	IL29	0,17	0,21	1,27
Siglec-5	0,63	0,87	1,37	MMP-10	0,05	0,08	1,51
BMP-7	not detect.	not detect.	not detect.	SAA	0,14	0,16	1,18
IL-18 BP alpha	0,14	0,09	0,65	Fcr RIIB/C	0,06	0,07	1,01
MMP-1	0,20	0,28	1,39	IL-31	0,05	0,08	1,64
TGF-alpha	0,12	0,10	0,85	NCAM-1	0,19	0,21	1,10
Cardiotrophin-1	not detect.	not detect.	not detect.	Siglec-9	0,06	0,05	0,84
IL-18 R beta	0,17	0,16	0,93	Ferritin	0,12	0,20	1,66
MMP-13	0,11	0,13	1,13	Insulin	0,10	0,07	0,65
TGF beta 2	0,19	0,21	1,13	Nidogen-1	0,26	0,30	1,16
CD14	0,36	0,57	1,55	TACE	0,06	0,10	1,58
MMP-3	0,08	0,20	2,58	FLRG	not detect.	not detect.	not detect.
MMP-9	0,10	0,20	1,93	Luteinizing Hormone	0,10	0,11	1,15
Tie-1	not detect.	not detect.	not detect.	NrCAM	0,08	0,11	1,30
CXCL-16	0,31	0,45	1,48	TIM-1	0,04	0,04	0,85
IL-2 R beta	0,11	0,18	1,73	Follistatin	0,14	0,15	1,04
MPIF-1	not detect.	not detect.	not detect.	LIMPII	0,03	0,04	1,20
Tie-2	0,06	0,08	1,31	NRG1-beta 1	0,13	0,12	0,92
DR6 (TNFRSF21)	0,12	0,15	1,18	TRAIL R2	0,13	0,10	0,80
IL-2 R gamma	0,12	0,13	1,13	ACE-2	not detect.	not detect.	not detect.
NGF R	not detect.	not detect.	not detect.	Cathepsin S	0,08	0,12	1,52
TIMP-4	0,22	0,28	1,30	DKK-3	0,06	0,06	1,09
beta IG-H3	0,09	0,08	0,82	HVEM	0,10	0,16	1,58
Cripto-1	not detect.	not detect.	not detect.	Alpha-Fetoprotein	not detect.	not detect.	not detect.
ErbB2	not detect.	not detect.	not detect.	CCL14a	0,06	0,12	2,13

PSA-free	0,04	0,05	1,08	DKK-4	0,04	0,05	1,23
CA125	0,03	0,05	1,45	IL-13R1	0,10	0,12	1,17
CRP	0,09	0,13	1,44	Angiopoietin-1	0,12	0,20	1,63
Erythropoietin R	not detect.	not detect.	not detect.	CCL21	0,15	0,30	2,03
S-100b	not detect.	not detect.	not detect.	DPPIV	0,14	0,32	2,32
CA15-3	0,04	0,06	1,42	IL-17B	not detect.	not detect.	not detect.
DAN	0,04	0,04	1,07	Angiostatin	0,08	0,10	1,19
FSH	0,13	0,12	0,92	CD23	0,10	0,11	1,05
Shh N	0,07	0,09	1,25	E-Cadherin	not detect.	not detect.	not detect.
CA19-9	0,06	0,07	1,22	IL-17C	0,06	0,09	1,43
Decorin	0,14	0,19	1,37	ANGPTL4	not detect.	not detect.	not detect.
HB-EGF	0,07	0,07	0,90	CD40 Ligand	0,03	0,06	1,87
Thyroglobulin	not detect.	not detect.	not detect.	EDA-A2	not detect.	not detect.	not detect.
4-1BB	0,05	0,05	0,95	IL-17F	0,03	0,05	1,51
Carbonic Anhydrase IX	not detect.	not detect.	not detect.	Bate2 M	0,17	0,33	1,88
DKK-1	not detect.	0,04	APO SN only	CEA	0,15	0,16	1,02
hCGa, intact	not detect.	not detect.	not detect.	EG-VEGF	0,11	0,19	1,81
Ubiquitin+1	0,04	0,05	1,20	IL-17R	0,06	0,08	1,31
BCMA	not detect.	not detect.	not detect.	EpCAM	not detect.	not detect.	not detect.
CEACAM-1	0,08	0,05	0,55	Procalcitonin	not detect.	not detect.	not detect.

Table 1 shows a semi-quantitative analysis of soluble factors found in the supernatant of irradiated apoptotitc and non-apoptotic cells.

Results of experiments investigating the cardioprotective properties of supernatants obtained from apoptotic PBMC[39]

Analysis of soluble factors detectable in cell culture supernatants of irradiated human PBMC (termed APOSEC^H)

In order to further determine the broad spectrum of soluble factors released by apoptotic cells we analysed the cell culture supernatant of irradiated cells by means of proteome membrane arrays and ELISA. As described previously, human PBMC were irradiated with 60 Gy and cells were incubated for 24 hours. After that incubation period, cell-free supernatants were harvested and analysed for cytokines, chemokines and growth factors that are associated with tissue repair mechanisms, angiogenesis, progenitor cell mobilization and homing to sites of injury.

To gain a better overview over the whole bandwidth of regenerative factors released by apoptotic cells, we screened the supernatants for cytokines and pro-angiogenic mediators using commercially available proteome membrane arrays.

A1,2: Positive control	B1,2: ---	C1,2: ---	D1,2: ---	E1,2: Positive control
A3,4: C5a	B3,4: IL-1a	C3,4: IL-10	D3,4: IL-32α	E3,4: RANTES
A5,6: CD40 ligand	B5,6: IL-1β	C5,6: IL-12 p70	D5,6: CXCL10	E5,6: CXCL12/SDF-1
A7,8: G-CSF	B7,8: IL-1ra	C7,8: IL-13	D7,8: CXCL11	E7,8: TNF-α
A9,10: GM-CSF	B9,10: IL-2	C9,10: IL-16	D9,10: MCP-1	E9,10: sTREM-1
A11,12: GRO-α	B11,12: IL-4	C11,12: IL-17	D11,12: MIF	E11,12: ---
A13,14: CCL1/I-309	B13,14: IL-5	C13,14: IL-17E	D13,14: MIP-1α	E13,14: ---
A15,16: sICAM-1	B15,16: IL-6	C15,16: IL-23	D15,16: MIP-1β	E15,16: ---
A17,18: IFN-γ	B17,18: IL-8	C17,18: IL-27	D17,18: PAI-1	E17,18: ---
A19-20: Positive control	B19,20: ---	C19,20: ---	D19-20: ---	E19,20: Negative control

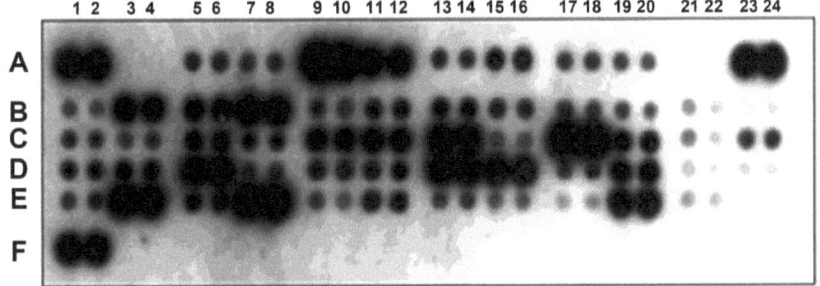

A1,2: Positive control	B1,2: TF	C1,2: GDNF	D1,2: MIP-1a	E1,2: Serpin B5	F1,2: Positive control
A3,4: ---	B3,4: CXCL16	C3,4: GM-CSF	D3,4: MMP-8	E3,4: PAI-1	F3,4: ---
A5,6: Activin A	B5,6: CD26	C5,6: HB-EGF	D5,6: MMP-9	E5,6: Serpin F1	F5,6: ---
A7,8: ADAMTS-1	B7,8: EGF	C7,8: HGF	D7,8: NRG1-β1	E7,8: TIMP-1	F7,8: ---
A9,10: Angiogenin	B9,10: EG-VEGF	C9,10: IGFBP-1	D9,10: Pentraxin 3	E9,10: TIMP-4	F9,10: ---
A11,12: Angiopoietin-1	B11,12: CD105	C11,12: IGFBP-2	D11,12: PD-ECGF	E11,12: TSP-1	F11,12: ---
A13,14: Angiopoietin-2	B13,14: Endostatin	C13,14: IGFBP-3	D13,14: PDGF-AA	E13,14: TSP-2	F13,14: ---
A15,16: Plasminogen	B15,16: Endothelin-1	C15,16: IL-1β	D15,16: PDGF-AB/BB	E15,16: uPA	F15,16: ---
A17,18: Amphiregulin	B17,18: FGF acidic	C17,18: IL-8	D17,18: Persephin	E17,18: Vasohibin	F17,18: ---
A19,20: Artemin	B19,20: FGF basic	C19,20: TGF-β1	D19,20: CXCL4	E19,20: VEGF	F19,20: ---
A21,22: ---	B21,22: FGF-4	C21,22: Leptin	D21,22: PlGF	E21,22: VEGF-C	F21,22: ---
A23,24: Positive control	B23,24: FGF-7	C23,24: MCP-1	D23,24: Prolactin	E23,24: ---	F23,24: Negative control

Figure 10 shows a semi-quantitative evaluation of soluble factors that are detectable in the supernatant of irradiated apoptotic cells.

As shown in Table 2, human PBMC secreted high amounts of various paracrine mediators. Compared to non-irradiated controls, higher concentrations of IL-8, GRO-alpha, ENA-78, RANTES, sICAM-1, MIF, VEGF, IL-1ra and IL-16 were detected in a cell density dependent fashion. In comparison to the aforementioned factors, little if any secretion was detected for factors such as MCP-1, IL-10, IGF-1, HGF, FGF-2, TGF-β, SDF-1, G-CSF and GM-CSF (see Table 2).

Analysis of soluble factors secreted by non-irradiated cells and irradiated apoptotic PBMC (APOSEC)

soluble factors (ng/ml)	viable PBMC			apoptotic PBMC			sig.
	$1·10^6$	$2.5·10^6$	$25·10^6$	$1·10^6$	$2.5·10^6$	$25·10^6$	
IL-8	1.74 ±0.40	1.93 ±0.09	10.49 ±3.53	1.22 ±0.29	2.30 ±0.13	18.01 ±2.87	ns ns ¥
GRO-alpha	0.17 ±0.09	0.36 ±0.09	2.06 ±1.58	0.07 ±0.02	0.48 ±0.09	3.95 ±0.93	ns ns ns
ENA-78	3.41 ±1.34	29.93 ±3.41	34.89 ±16.33	3.93 ±1.43	37.86 ±12.73	108.86 ±27.88	ns ns ¥
MCP-1	1.66 ±0.65	0.47 ±0.21	0.27 ±0.00	0.76 ±0.19	0.74 ±0.17	0.27 ±0.00	ns ns ns
RANTES	8.32 ±0.18	18.62 ±3.21	37.63 ±2.72	4.01 ±0.05	22.25 ±3.64	51.58 ±4.44	ns ns ns
HMGB1	0.63 ±0.39	3.44 ±2.11	33.57 ±6.45	2.74 ±0.27	6.46 ±1.12	20.51 ±3.62	† ns ns
MMP9	4.14 ±0.91	14.59 ±2.75	29.46 ±8.29	0.99 ±0.16	3.61 ±0.59	19.35 ±5.34	† ‡ ns
sICAM-1	0.14 ±0.04	1.43 ±0.25	7.43 ±0.85	0.42 ±0.25	2.09 ±0.42	9.40 ±1.29	ns ns ¥
VEGF165	0.13 ±0.01	0.42 ±0.04	0.82 ±0.34	0.15 ±0.02	0.64 ±0.04	4.39 ±1.22	ns ns ¥
MIF	4.84 ±0.09	17.79 ±0.95	13.24 ±0.85	5.85 ±0.22	20.15 ±1.14	58.99 ±1.17	ns ns ¥
PAI-1	1.25 ±0.35	1.93 ±0.29	49.60 ±9.04	0.00 ±0.00	5.06 ±3.25	45.86 ±1.43	ns ns ns
IL-16	0.0 ±0.0	0.11 ±0.02	0.84 ±0.31	0.00 ±0.00	1.25 ±0.07	5.25 ±0.52	ns ‡ ns
IL-1ra	0.35 ±0.09	0.52 ±0.17	2.16 ±0.96	0.13 ±0.04	0.41 ±0.17	6.43 ±1.33	ns ns ¥
IL-10	0.01 ±0.00	0.00 ±0.0	0.05 ±0.01	0.02 ±0.01	0.02 ±0.01	0.06 ±0.01	ns ns ns
IGF-I	0.00 ±0.00	0.01 ±0.0	0.03 ±0.02	0.00 ±0.00	0.01 ±0.01	0.03 ±0.03	ns ns ns
HGF	0.33 ±0.08	0.16 ±0.01	0.69 ±0.19	0.11 ±0.03	0.07 ±0.02	0.79 ±0.19	ns ns ns
FGF-2	0.56 ±0.02	0.53 ±0.00	0.59 ±0.01	0.48 ±0.01	0.53 ±0.02	0.55 ±0.02	ns ns ns
TGF-β	0.08 ±0.01	0.10 ±0.01	0.21 ±0.07	0.06 ±0.01	0.09 ±0.02	0.39 ±0.09	ns ns ns
SDF-1	0.17 ±0.0	0.19 ±0.0	0.22 ±0.03	0.16 ±0.01	0.15 ±0.07	0.12 ±0.04	ns ns ns
G-CSF	0.00 ±0.00	0.00 ±0.00	0.00 ±0.00	0.00 ±0.00	0.00 ±0.00	0.00 ±0.00	ns ns ns
GM-CSF	0.00 ±0.00	0.00 ±0.00	0.07 ±0.02	0.00 ±0.00	0.00 ±0.00	0.08 ±0.02	ns ns ns

Table 2: Analysis of soluble factors secreted by non-irradiated cells and irradiated apoptotic PBMC (APOSEC).
Cells were incubated in three different cell concentrations for 24 hours. Supernatants were analyzed for cytokines, chemokines and growth factors (n=5). † p<0.05 $1·10^6$ viable PBMC vs. $1·10^6$ apoptotic PBMC, ‡ p<0.05 $2.5·10^6$ viable PBMC vs. $2.5·10^6$ apoptotic PBMC, ¥ p<0.05 $25·10^6$ viable PBMC vs. $25·10^6$ apoptotic PBMC.

Up-regulation of anti-apoptotic and cytoprotective factors by supernatants of apoptotic cells

Based on the finding that irradiated apoptotic cells secreted a vast spectrum of cytokines and growth factors, we sought to investigate whether these mediators have a direct influence on cardiac myocytes. For these purpose, human cardiomyocytes were incubated together with APOSEC^H in different concentrations. In order to gain an overview which anti-apoptotic or cytoprotective factors are involved in these mechanisms, we utilized a proteome membrane array (see Figure 11).

Apoptosis Array

A1,2: pos con	B1,2: Bad	C1,2: TRAIL R17DR4	D1,2: PON2	E1,2: pos con
A3,4: ---	B3,4: Bax	C3,4: TRAIL R2/DR5	D3,4: P21/CIP1	E3,4: ---
A5,6: ---	B5,6: Bcl-2	C5,6: FADD	D5,6: P27/Kip1	E5,6: ---
A7,8: ---	B7,8: Bcl-x	C7,8: Fas/TNFRSF6	D7,8: Phospho-p53 (S15)	E7,8: ---
A9,10: ---	B9,10: Pro-Caspase-3	C9,10: HIF-1alpha	D9,10: Phospho-p53 (S46)	E9,10: ---
A11,12: ---	B11,12: Cleaved Caspase-3	C11,12: HO-1/HSP32	D11,12: Phospho-p53 (S392)	E11,12: ---
A13,14: ---	B13,14: Catalase	C13,14: HO-2	D13,14: Phospho-Rad17	E13,14: ---
A15,16: ---	B15-16: cIAP-1	C15,16: HSP27	D15,16: SMAC/Diablo	E15,16: ---
A17,18: ---	B17,18: c-IAP-2	C17,18: HSP60	D17,18: Survivin	E17,18: ---
A19,20: ---	B19,20: Claspin	C19,20: HSP70	D19-20: TNF RI/TNFRSF1A	E19,20: ---
A21,22: ---	B21,22: Clusterin	C21,22: HTRA2/Omi	D21,22: XIAP	E21,22: ---
A23-24: Pos con	B23,24: Cytochrome c	C23,24: Livin	D23,24: PBS	E23,24: ---

Figure 11 Membrane array analysis for apoptosis related proteins regulated by APOSEC[H] in human primary cardiac myocytes. As shown, mainly Bcl-2 and Heat shock proteins were up-regulated after exposure to APOSEC[H].

To verify the results obtained by proteome membrane array analysis, Western Blot assays were performed to evaluate up-regulation of the anti-apoptotic and cytoprotective factors Bcl-2 and BAG1[47, 48].

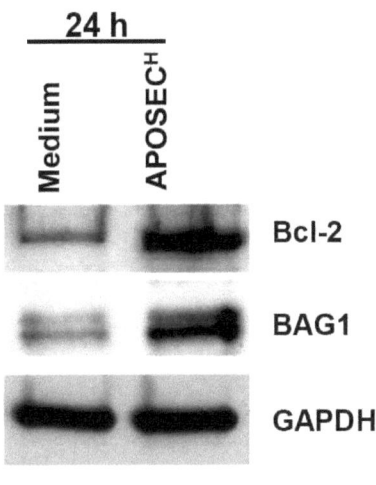

Figure 12 Expression of Bcl-2 and BAG1 in human cardiac myocytes after APOSEC treatment. 24 hours after start of co-incubation, expression of the anti-apoptotic proteins Bcl-2 and BAG1 was analysed by Western blotting. Proteins were normalized to the house-keeping gene GAPDH.

Furthermore, we investigated effects of APOSEC treatment on the triggering of signalling factors that were associated with cardioprotective mechanisms and cardiac (ischaemic) pre- and post-conditioning, e.g. AKT, Erk1/2, CREB and Heat shock protein 27 (Hsp27) [49-56].

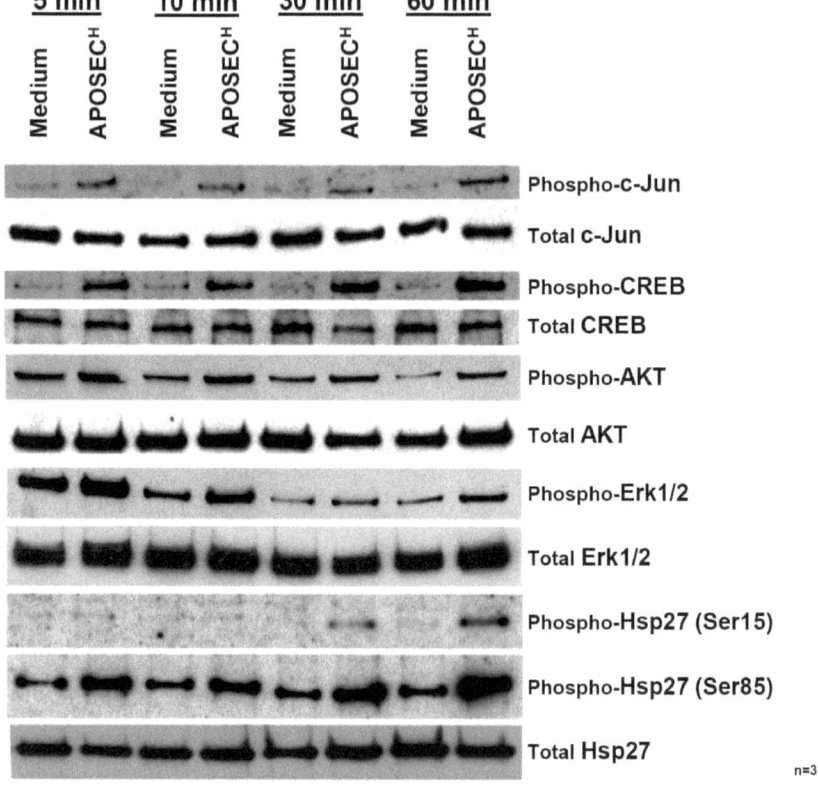

Figure 13 Human cardiac myocytes were treated with APOSEC[H], cell extracts were prepared after the indicated time intervals. Western Blot analysis shows increased phosphorylation of c-Jun, CREB, AKT, Erk1/2 and Hsp27.

In order to test a dose-dependent relationship of APOSEC treatment and the induction of cardioprotective signalling factors, further Western Blot assays were conducted.

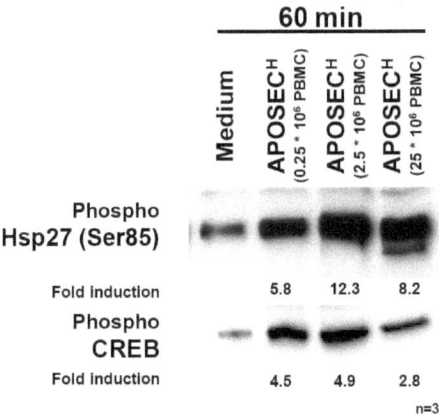

Figure 14 shows a dose-dependent increase in phosphorylation of Hsp27 and CREB. Highest levels were achieved when cardiac myocytes were incubated with APOSEC derived from $2.5 \cdot 10^6$ apoptotic PBMC. Even APOSEC obtained from just $0.25 \cdot 10^6$ apoptotic PBMC potently induced the phosphorylation of Hsp27 and CREB.

Moreover, we sought to determine whether APOSEC treatment confers direct cell protection to stressed cardiomyocytes. For this purpose, we utilized a cell starvation/ growth factor withdrawal assay of human cardiac myocytes. When APOSEC was added to these cultures in increasing concentrations, a dose-dependent effect was observed.

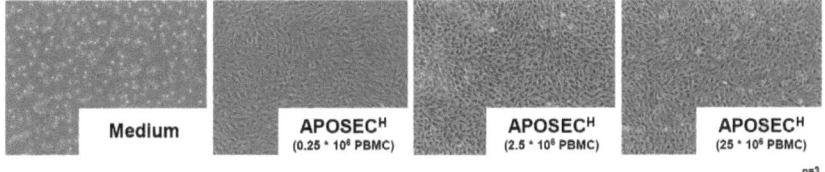

Figure 15 shows that growth factor withdrawal reduces cell viability of human cardiac myocytes. When APOSEC was added in increasing doses, cell viability was restored again.

APOSEC treatment in a rat model of AMI

Based on these *in vitro* findings that APOSEC up-regulates cytoprotective factors and increases survival of human cardiac myocytes, we sought to investigate intravenous APOSEC administration in a small animal model of acute myocardial infarction by ligation of the left anterior descending artery (LAD). The injection of fresh cell culture medium or supernatants obtained from non-irradiated viable cells served as controls in this experimental setting.

Three days after induction of AMI and injection of APOSEC^R, fresh medium or supernatants of non-irradiated cells, rat hearts were explanted, fixed in formalin solution and analysed microscopically by means of histology (H&E staining). Compared to the two control groups, hearts of APOSEC^R injected animals evidenced less myocardial damage and also less signs of cellular infiltration in the ischaemic areas of the myocardium.

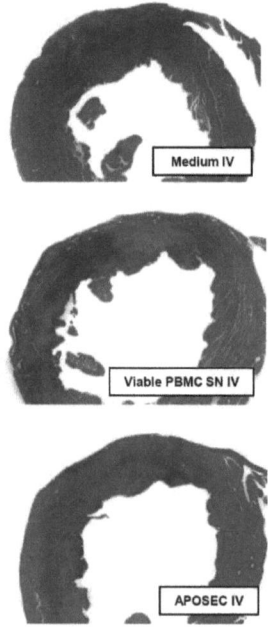

Figure 16 shows representative images of rat hearts three days after AMI. Hearts from APOSEC^R injected animals show less immune cell infiltrates and myocardial damage.

Image J software was used to quantify the extent of myocardial necrosis by means of planimetry. Animals that were injected with fresh cell culture medium showed a mean area of necrosis of 20.56% ±1.71 (SEM, expressed as % of the left ventricle). Rats with injection of supernatants derived from non-irradiated viable cells evidenced mean values of 21.08% ±2.76. This damage was reduced to 10.81% ±2.58 in animals that were treated with APOSEC derived from rat cells (p=0.017 and 0.03 vs. controls).

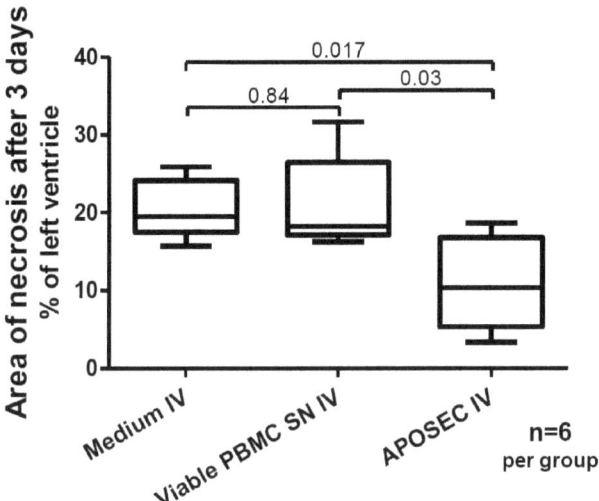

Figure 17 shows results obtained by planimetry three days after induction of AMI.

In accordance with our previous results (injection of cell suspensions of apoptotic PBMC after AMI) we found denser cellular infiltrates in the ischaemic myocardium of APOSEC treated animals compared to the two control groups.

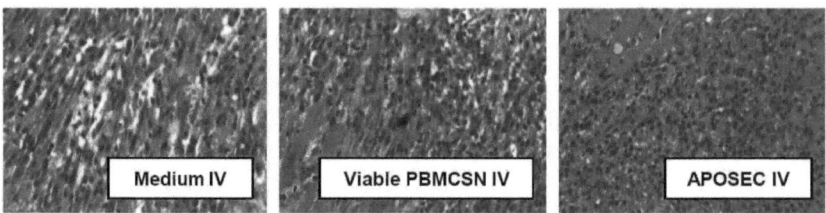

Figure 18 shows H&E-stained specimens of rat myocardium three days after induction of AMI. The cellular infiltrate in the ischaemic myocardium appears to be much more consolidated in APOSEC^R injected animals.

Immunohistology was utilized to further characterize the cellular infiltrate in the ischaemic myocardium. Myocardial specimens obtained three days after AMI were analysed for the markers CD68 and c-kit as cell populations bearing these epitopes were also enriched in rats that were injected with suspensions of apoptotic PBMC (see previous results).

In accordance, higher levels of infiltrating cells staining positive for CD68 were detected in specimens of rats that were injected with APOSEC^R. In total, 60.8 ±4.8 positive cells per high power field (HPF) were found in controls, 75.6 ±7.6 in rats injected with supernatants of non-irradiated cells and 114.2 ±11.6 in animals that were treated with APOSEC^R.

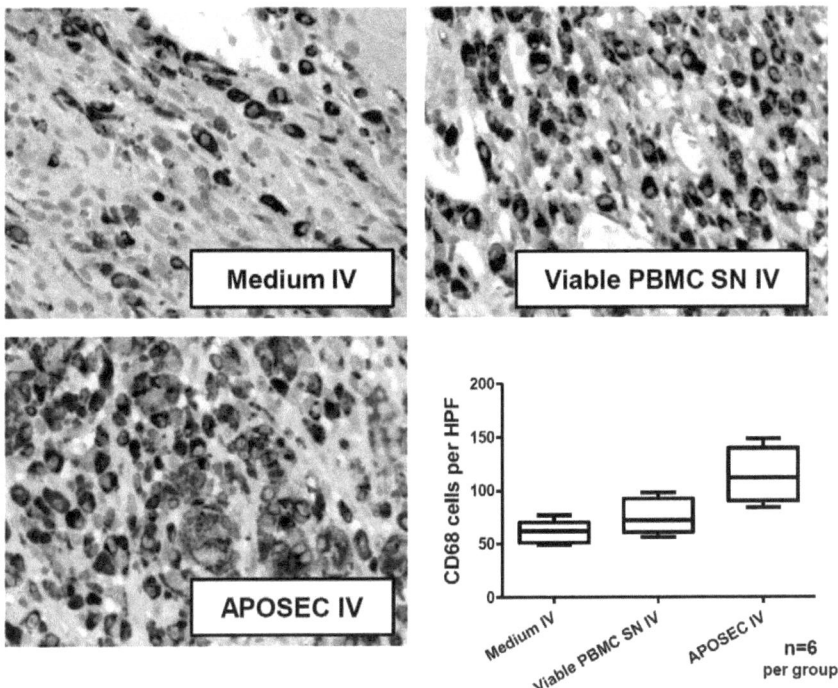

Figure 19 shows immunohistological images of specimens stained for the marker CD68 and a boxplot analysis of the obtained results.

Moreover, an immunohistological analysis was conducted for the marker c-kit. In our previous experiments, higher numbers of cells bearing that marker were found in the epicardial regions of animals that were injected with apoptotic cells. A similar result was found in rats that were treated with APOSEC.

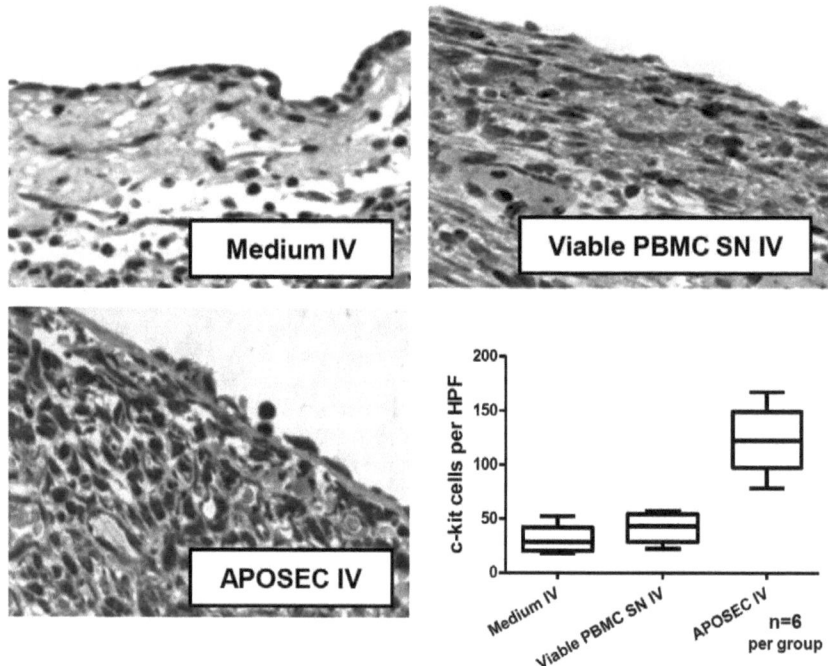

Figure 20 shows immunohistological staining for the marker c-kit and a boxplot analysis of the obtained data.

Only a few positive cells were found in myocardial specimens of control animals and rats injected with supernatants of non-irradiated cells with mean levels of 30.4 ±5.9 and 41.6 ±6.1 cells per HPF. In APOSEC^R injected rats, these levels increased to 123.0 ±14.3 c-kit positive cells in epicardial regions of the infarcted myocardium.

After homogenisation of cardiac specimens, the quantity of c-kit and CD68 positive cells was also determined by flow cytometry. Both cell populations were enriched in APOSEC^R-injected animals, as evidenced by a mean increase of 37% of CD68 cells and of 107% of c-kit positive cells compared to control animals

In order to investigate medium to long term results of APOSEC treatment in regards to ventricular remodelling, a second subgroup of animals was scarified six weeks after induction of AMI by LAD ligation.

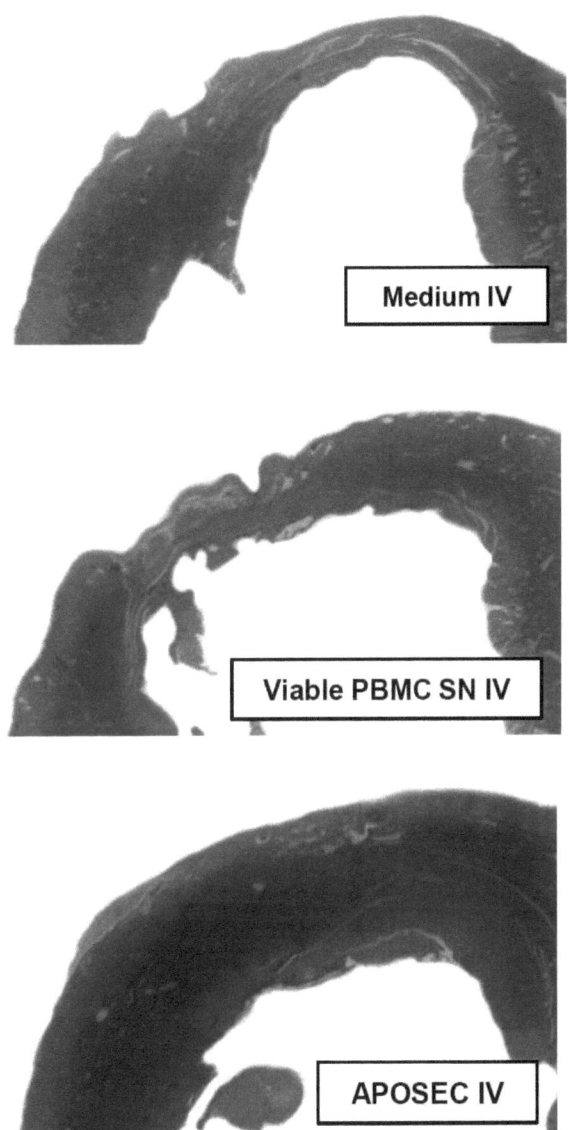

Figure 21 shows myocardial specimens obtained six weeks after induction of AMI. Hearts of APOSEC treated rats evidence less scar formation and less ventricular remodelling compared to controls.

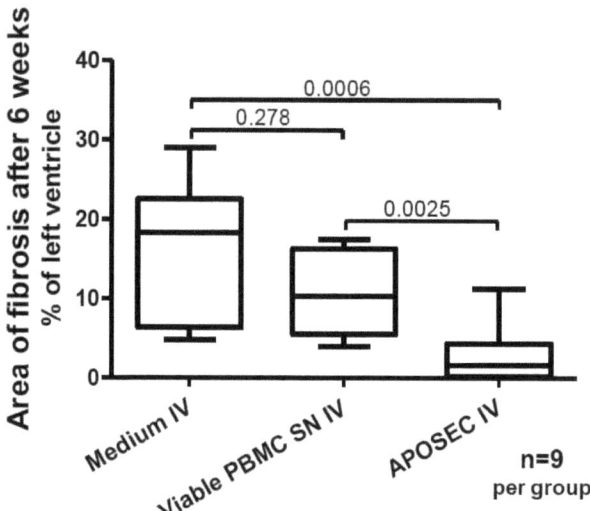

Figure 22 shows results obtained by planimetric analysis of rat heart specimens stained according to an Elastics van Gieson protocol. Results indicate a significant reduction of scar area compared to controls.

Assessment of cardiac function by means of echocardiography

In order to document functional changes of cardiac function after AMI induction, echocardiography was utilized and values of ejection fraction (EF), shortening fraction (SF), left ventricular end-diastolic diameter (LVEDD) and left ventricular end-systolic diameters (LVESD) were recorded.

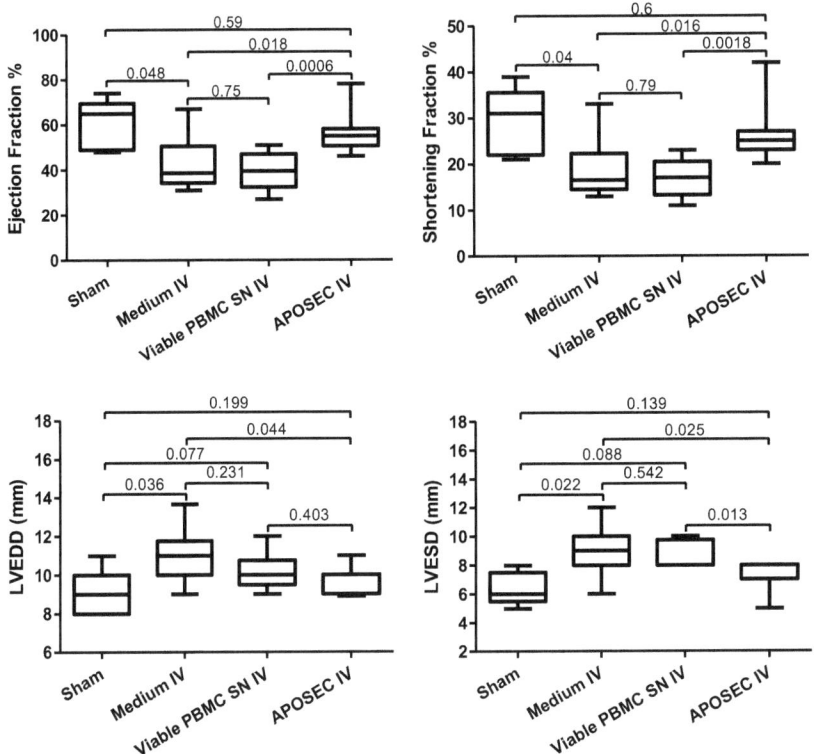

Figure 23 shows results obtained by echocardiography six weeks after LAD ligation and induction of AMI. Functional parameters of the heart (EF, SF, LVEDD, LVESD) were improved in APOSEC injected animals in comparison to medium or viable cell supernatant injected rats.

Six weeks after induction of AMI, the mean ejection fractions (EF), shortening fractions (SF), left ventricular end-diastolic diameter (LVEDD) and left ventricular end-systolic diameter (LVESD) were determined to be 43.04%±4.17 (EF), 19.00%±2.29 (SF), 10.96mm±0.51 (LVEDD) and 9.00mm±0.63 (LVESD) in animals that were injected with culture medium alone and 39.38%±2.89 (EF), 16.88%±1.45 (SF), 10.17mm±0.33 (LVEDD) and 8.63mm±0.32 (LVESD) in rats which were injected with the supernatants of non-irradiated viable PBMC. Interestingly, APOSEC injected rats evidenced significantly improved functional parameters: 56.22%±3.05 (LVEF; p=0.018 vs. medium and p=0.0006 vs. viable cell supernatants),

26.33%±2.11 (SF; p=0.016 vs. medium and p=0.0018 vs. viable cell supernatants), 9.77mm±0.23 (LVEDD; p=0.044 vs. medium) and 7.33mm±0.33 (LVESD; p=0.025 vs. medium and p=0.013 vs. viable cell supernatants). Mean levels of cardiac function of healthy animals without induction of myocardial infarction (sham operation) were as follows: 60.40%±4.95 (LVEF), 29.20%±3.26 (SF), 9.00mm±0.55 (LVEDD) and 6.40mm±0.51 (LVESD).

Large animal AMI model

Based on these results obtained *in vitro* and in small animal experiments, we set up a large animal experiment of closed chest reperfused myocardial infarction using a porcine model investigating the therapeutic potential of APOSEC. For this purpose, APOSEC^P was administered 40 minutes after onset of myocardial ischaemia in two different doses, in a low dose group with reconstituted cell culture supernatants obtained from $250 \cdot 10^6$ apoptotic PBMC and in a high dose group with supernatants obtained from $1 \cdot 10^9$ apoptotic PBMC.

For a short term analysis of the cardioprotective effects induced by APOSEC^P treatment, a subgroup of animals was sacrificed 24 hours after reperfused myocardial infarction. The explanted hearts were evaluated using a staining protocol of tetrazolium cloride (TTC) and Evans blue solution. Necrotic myocardial tissue remained unstained.

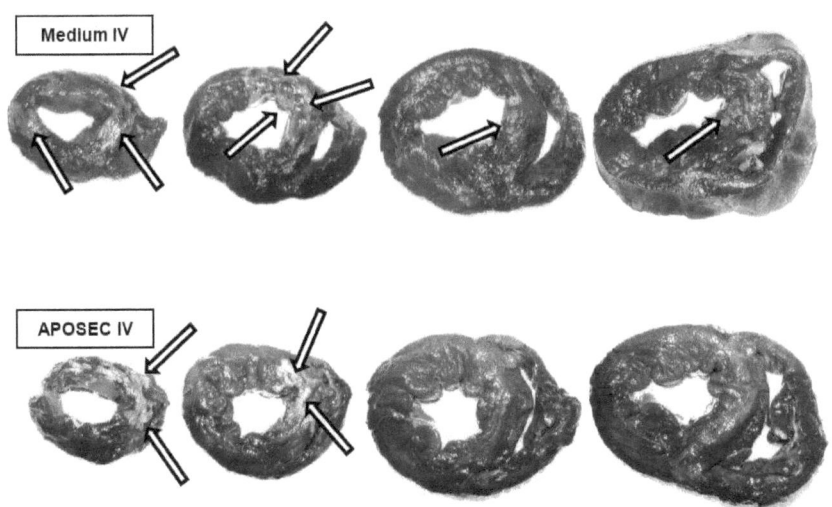

Figure 24 shows representative images of porcine hearts explanted 24 hours after reperfused myocardial infarction stained with tetrazolium chloride (TTC) and Evans blue solution. Arrows indicate necrotic tissue

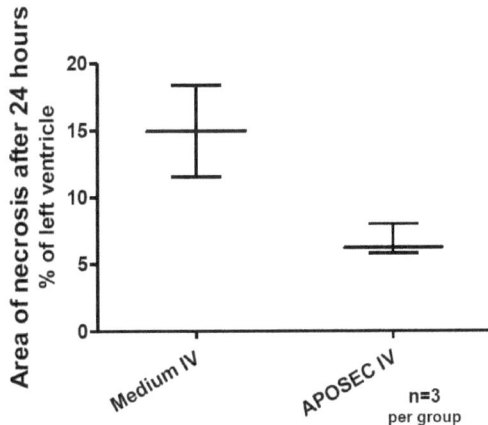

Figure 25 shows results obtained by a planimetric analysis of porcine hearts demonstrating a reduction of myocardial injury by APOSEC^P treatment after 24 hours.

In order to determine the reduction of myocardial injury by APOSEC treatment, an ELISA assay investigating Troponin I release over the first 24 hours after AMI was conducted.

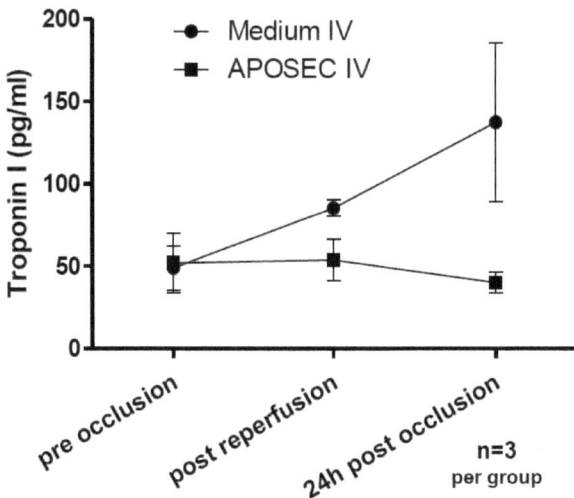

Figure 26 shows that plasma Troponin I levels of APOSEC^P infused pigs remained at base line whereas an increase was detected in medium injected control animals.

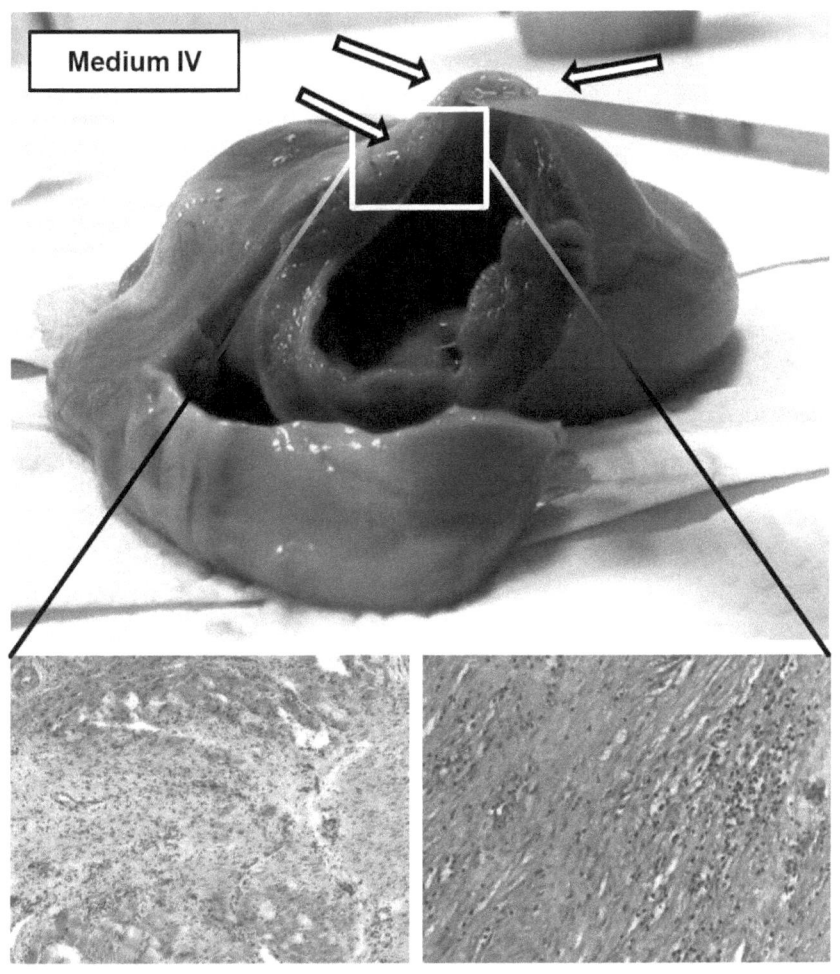

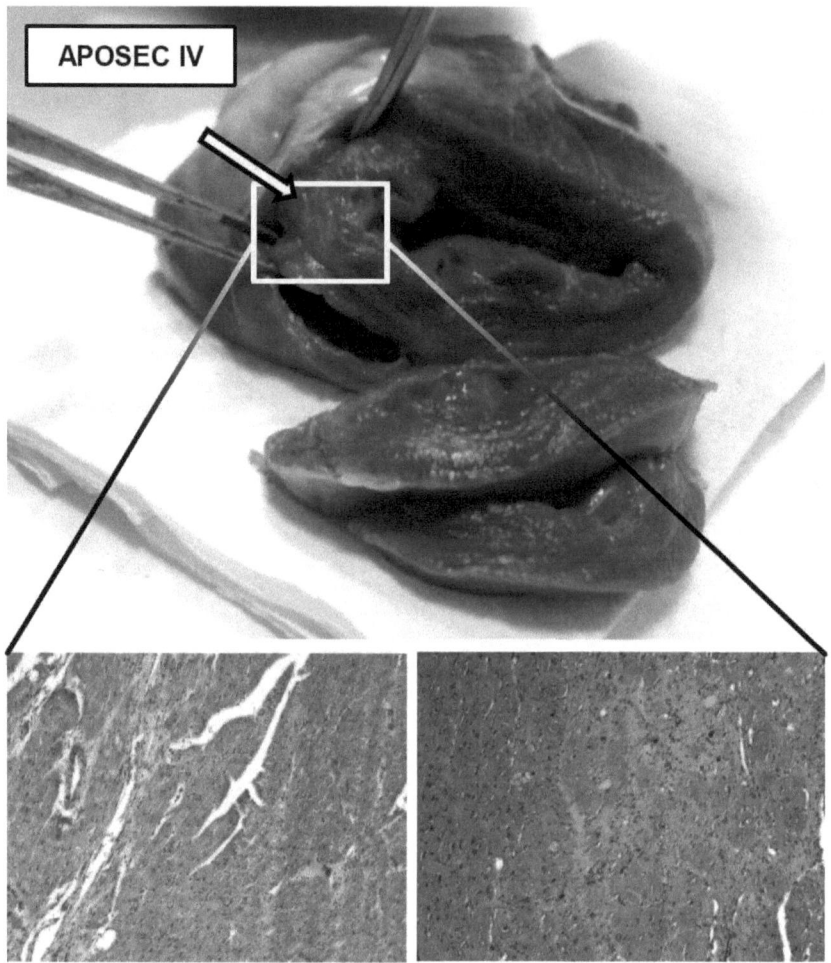

Figure 27 shows representative images of porcine hearts explanted 30 days after AMI. Hearts of APOSEC^P-injected pigs evidenced only very marginal scar tissue formation in the myocardium compared to control animals (Medium IV) where large infarcts were common. H&E-stained and Movat's pentachrome-stained specimens of the infarcted myocardium shown in the lower part of the figure indicate less signs of collagen deposition and more viable cardiomyocytes within the scar tissue of the left ventricle compared to control animals.

Cardiac MRI evaluation 3 and 30 days after AMI

	Parameters	Medium control (n=8)	250·10⁶ apoptotic PBMC (low dose APOSEC, n=7)	1·10⁹ apoptotic PBMC (high dose APOSEC, n=7)
after 3 days	weight (kg)	31.86 ±9.1	30.86 ±1.6 ns	33.33 ±1.3 ns
	age (days)	90 ±0	90 ±0 ns	90 ±0 ns
	LVEDV (ml)	67.59 ±2.7	64.19 ±5.4 ns	63.73 ±1.6 ns
	LVESV (ml)	38.42 ±2.5	35.96 ±3.0 ns	33.93 ±2.1 ns
	LVSV (ml)	29.17 ±1.3	28.23 ±3.2 ns	29.77 ±1.8 ns
	LVEF (%)	43.38 ±1.9	43.63 ±2.8 ns	46.65 ±2.9 ns
	HR/min.	111 ±6	109 ±5 ns	111 ±13 ns
	CO (l/min.)	3.24 ±0.1	3.03 ±0.3 ns	3.28 ±0.3 ns
	CI (l/min/m²)	3.64 ±0.1	3.59 ±0.4 ns	3.82 ±0.4 ns
	Infarct %	18.17 ±1.7	14.01 ±1.9 ns	8.66 ±1.5 **
after 30 days	weight (kg)	39.43 ±0.5	37.00 ±1.9 ns	48.83 ±0.7 ***
	age (days)	120 ±0	120 ±0 ns	120 ±0 ns
	LVEDV (ml)	54.74 ±4.1	53.43 ±3.2 ns	65.99 ±3.5 ns
	LVESV (ml)	32.93 ±4.0	31.89 ±2.9 ns	28.71 ±3.5 ns
	LVSV (ml)	21.84 ±1.8	21.54 ±1.9 ns	37.29 ±1.7 ***
	LVEF (%)	40.54 ±3.6	40.64 ±3.2 ns	57.05 ±3.3 **
	HR/min.	114 ±7	108 ±7 ns	107 ±5 ns
	CO (l/min.)	2.44 ±0.1	2.28 ±0.1 ns	3.98 ±0.2 ***
	CI (l/min/m²)	2.46 ±0.1	2.40 ±0.1 ns	3.51 ±0.2 ***
	Infarct %	12.60 ±1.3	11.50 ±1.5 ns	6.92 ±1.4 *

ns   no significance versus control
*   p<0.05 versus control
**   p<0.01 versus control
***   p<0.001 versus control

Table 3 shows parameters obtained three and 30 days after reperfused myocardial infarction. Cardiac MRI analysis was conducted and parameters of cardiac function were obtained from pigs treated with low and high dose APOSEC and from control animals that were infused with reconstituted cell culture medium (left ventricular end-diastolic diameter, LVEDD; left ventricular end-systolic diameter, LVESD; left ventricular stroke volume, LVSV; left ventricular ejection fraction, LVEF; heart rate, HR; cardiac index, CI; cardiac output, CO).

BARI score evaluations

In order to determine that all animals evidenced a comparable perfusion of the myocardium prior to occlusion of the LAD and a comparable extent of myocardium at risk, a modified BARI score was calculated based on angiographic images of the LAD the left circumflex artery (LCX). No significant differences were detected between the three groups.

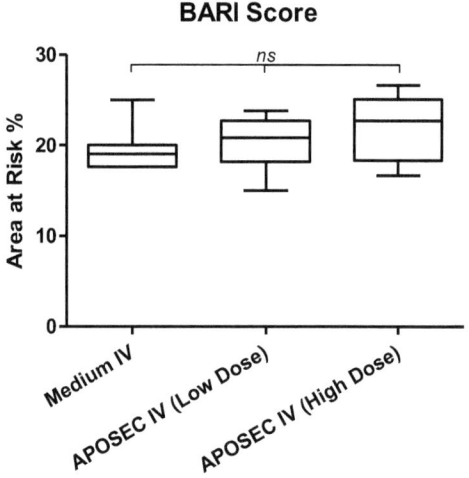

Figure 28 shows results obtained by BARI score calculation, no significant differences were observed between groups.

Discussion

Over the last decades, clinical research in cardiovascular medicine has focused on establishing early reperfusion after occlusion of a coronary artery and by doing so salvaging myocardium at risk for ischaemic cell death. Nevertheless, current treatment strategies do not address the key problem of myocardial ischaemia which is the loss of viable myocardium, composed of cardiomyocytes, vascular cells, and connective tissue cells. The consequence of this loss of vital contractile tissue is that patients continue to experience frequent hospitalisation after AMI and in many cases develop signs of heart failure.

Due to the detrimental processes associated with ischaemic tissue injury, great hopes were put in stem cell research and its clinical application for cardiovascular medicine. Although small animal experiments investigating the regenerative potential of stem cell therapy evidenced very convincing results, clinical trials showed only moderately beneficial effects results compared to control patients or these effects lasted only for a short period of time [11, 12].

Based on the hypothesis stated by Thum and Anker *et al.* [15] that apoptotic stem cells transplanted after AMI might modulate the inflammatory response and prevent ventricular remodelling, we sought to prove this in *in vitro* and *in vivo* experiments. Instead of bone marrow cells we used the more easily obtainable "cellular material" of PBMC based on two assumptions: first, the beneficial potential bone marrow cells, peripheral blood cells or their supernatants can be assumed to be of no major difference [31] and second, in order to promote the clinical application of cell therapy after AMI using easier obtainable cell types we have focused on PBMC instead of stem/progenitor cells. In our previous work we showed that apoptotic PBMC evidenced immunomodulatory effects *in vitro* and preserved cardiac function after AMI in a small animal model [22]. Based on these results we sought to further investigate how apoptotic cells prevent ventricular remodelling after AMI. Furthermore, we investigated additional ways of cell administration (i.e. intravenously and intramyocardially). Again, we found higher numbers of macrophages and cells expressing the markers c-kit and VEGF receptor 2 three days after AMI. This seems to be a pivotal point, as macrophages mediate the changeover from the initial phase of AMI to tissue stabilization, indicating a faster healing process within the ischaemic myocardium. This phenomenon of cell accumulation was detectable even to a much greater extent when the irradiated apoptotic cells where injected directly into the ischaemic tissue by intramyocardial injection. Another major finding was the fact that the treatment with apoptotic PBMC suspensions also reduced the extent of infarct dimension in this experimental AMI model. This reduced loss of vital myocardial also correlated with improved functional parameters in echocardiography. Animals injected with irradiated apoptotic cell suspensions evidenced a significant improvement of all tested parameters of cardiac function (ejection fraction, shortening fraction, ventricular diameters and volumes).

When analysing the composition of the extracellular matrix of the cardiac tissue, it was also of great interest that the configuration of the fibrotic scar was evidently altered in animals injected with apoptotic cells compared to controls. In specimens stained according to the Elastica van Gieson protocol, a considerable accumulation of elastic fibres especially in the border zone between vital cardiomyocytes and the fibrotic scar was detected. This alteration in the ratio of elastic and collagenous fibres could be a major factor contributing to the improvement of cardiac function parameters in rats injected with apoptotic cells. This was even more pronounced when these cell suspensions of apoptotic PBMC were injected directly into the ischaemic myocardium.

Due to this interesting finding, we sought to further investigate which factor might be accountable for the increased expression of elastic fibres. In the cellular infiltrate in the ischaemic myocardium of animals injected with suspension of apoptotic PBMC, higher numbers of cells staining positively for Insulin-like growth factor I (IGF-I) and Fibroblast growth factor 2 (FGF-2) were found in an immunohistological analysis. It has been reported that these two growth factors contribute directly to the synthesis of elastic fibres within the extracellular matrix and also regulate cardiac repair mechanisms after AMI [57-61]. There are a number of possible mechanisms by which a more favourable ratio of elastic and collagenous fibres in the cardiac scar tissue could delay the onset of ventricular dysfunction and remodelling after AMI. A cardiac scar tissue showing more elastic properties and being more resistant could function as a kind of shock absorbing cushion that might reduce the tractile effects on the scar tissue during systole. The recoil of the elastic fibres within the scar could provide a portion of passive energy that returns the scar size to pre-systolic dimensions. These mechanistic characteristic are important for preventing or reducing the risk for ventricular remodelling and by doing so might serve as an explanation for the preservation cardiac function in this experimental setting [62, 63].

Based on these convincing results we sought to further investigate the mechanisms of cardioprotective effects induced by apoptotic cells. When performing proteome membrane analysis in order to define the secretome of irradiated apoptotic PBMC compared to non-irradiated cells, an up-regulation of many pro-angiogenic cytokines, chemokines and growth factors was found. These findings also correlated with the results obtained in our previous study where we could show that irradiation and induction of apoptosis induced the expression of IL-8 and MMP9 transcripts in RT-PCR [22].

There has been a shift of opinion in the field of regenerative medicine since recent publications showed that soluble factors secreted by bone marrow cells during cell culture initiated proliferation and migration of coronary artery endothelial cells, endothelial tube formation and cell sprouting in a mouse aortic ring assay. Interestingly, supernatants obtained from peripheral blood cells showed no major differences in their potential to induce cell proliferation or to confer cytoprotective signalling [31]. In another publication it was shown that endothelial progenitor cell conditioned medium (termed EPC-CM) increased the formation of capillary outgrowth in a rat aortic ring model and enhanced the survival of serum-starved HUVEC [33]. The protective effects of EPC-CM were also demonstrated in an ischaemic hind limb model. The injection of EPC-CM increased the blood flow, muscle mitochondrial activity and also functional improvement in this experimental setting. More recently, the research group of Kalka showed that EPC-CM increased the resistance of HUVEC to oxidative stress by inducing anti-oxidative enzymes. Moreover, the resistance to stimuli inducing apoptosis *in vitro* was increased as well as cells showed an increased expression of the anti-apoptotic factor Bcl-2. Based on these results the authors concluded that EPC-CM contains cytoprotective proteins that confer anti-apoptotic and cytoprotective effects to stressed cells. Interestingly, the neutralization of factors found in the conditioned medium of EPC such as VEGF, IL-8 and MMP9 did not significantly reverse the cytoprotective effect of the EPC-CM. They argued that EPC secrete a broad bandwidth of factors which can cause many synergistic effects and may exert strong cytoprotective properties by increasing cellular anti-oxidant enzymes and increase the expression of pro-survival genes.

The mechanism described for cell culture supernatants obtained from bone marrow cells or (stressed) EPC shows many similarities to APOSEC. Here we could show that the conditioned culture medium obtained from irradiated apoptotic PBMC (APOSEC) induces cytoprotective mechanisms in cultured cardiomyocytes and protected them from starvation induced cell death. However, in contrary to the production of bone marrow cell derived supernatants, which requires a bone marrow biopsy, or the generation of EPC-CM, which requires rather elaborate laboratory techniques to expand these cell types, PBMC can be obtained quite simply from venous whole blood via venal puncture.

Due to the fact that the loss of vital myocardial tissue was significantly reduced three days after AMI in both animal models, we hypothesized that the main mechanism of action of APOSEC is in fact cytoprotection. This was substantiated by *in vitro* experiments, the incubation of human cardiac myocytes with APOSEC induced a rapid activation of several important survival factors described in the literature for cardioprotection and cardiac pre- and port-conditioning such as AKT, Erk1/2, p38 MAPK (all part of the ischaemia reperfusion injury salvage kinase pathway, RISK), c-JUN, cAMP-response element binding protein (CREB) and Hsp27 [56, 64, 65]. Moreover, Bcl-2 and BAG1, two major anti-apoptotic mediators were up-regulated in human cardiomyocytes exposed to APOSEC within 24 hours of cell culture.

Prompt restoration of coronary perfusion within the shortest time is currently considered to be the optimal standard of cardiac care for patients suffering from ST-elevation myocardial infarction (STEMI) according to the guidelines issued by the European Society of Cardiology and the American Heart Association (AHA) [66, 67]. In order to test the applicability of APOSEC infusions we implemented a closed chest large animal model of reperfused AMI which shows the most similarities to the clinical scenario AMI in human patients. In addition to this experimental simulation of standardized treatment of AMI in humans, APOSEC infusions were administered 40 minutes after the start of the LAD balloon occlusion. To further demonstrate a dose dependent response, APOSEC was administered in two different concentrations, i.e. resuspended lyophilised supernatants obtained from $1 \cdot 10^9$ and $250 \cdot 10^6$ apoptotic PBMC. The time intervals of 40 minutes until intravenous administration of APOSEC and 90 minutes until reperfusion were selected to accord with the clinical scenario of earliest possible intravenous therapy with approximately 30 - 40 minutes delay from symptom onset to diagnosis of AMI and start of intravenous therapy and 90 minutes until primary coronary intervention (PCI) and reperfusion. Short (three days) and long term (30 days) MRI results evidenced that one single (high dose) infusion of APOSEC led to a significant improvement of cardiac function and to a significant reduction of infarct dimension. Administration of low dose APOSEC evidences only marginally improved functional values compared to controls indicating a dose-dependent effect of this treatment.

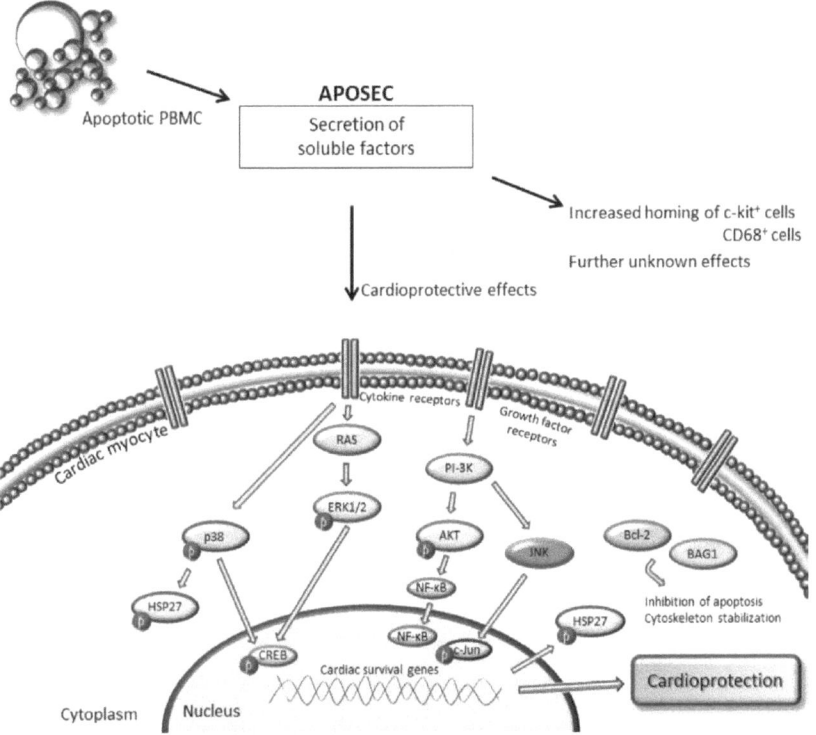

Figure 29 shows an illustration of the proposed mechanism of action that is induced by APOSEC treatment.

Conclusion

We demonstrated that cell culture supernatants of irradiated apoptotic PBMC can serve as an important therapeutic adjunct in the setting of AMI. Of major relevance is the fact that these supernatants containing soluble factor released by apoptotic cells can be lyophilised and stored as a powdery compound. The process of lyophilisation can increase the practicability of this therapeutic compound. In the clinical scenario of AMI, APOSEC preparations can be reconstituted in physiological saline solution and can be administered just like conventional intravenous infusion therapy. Comparable blood derived products such as intravenous immunoglobulin (IVIG) or coagulation factors have confirmed their clinical usefulness over the last decades [68-72]. Compared to these derivatives, APOSEC is a product made of soluble factors secreted by irradiated PBMC. This "biological" combines the following clinically favourable features: a) an easily obtainable cell material (PBMC) for production of APOSEC via venous blood withdrawal; b) low antigenicity due the cell-free nature of APOSEC and c) "off the shelf" use of APOSEC in the clinical setting of AMI requiring only intravenous administration in contrast to previous clinical trials investigating stem cells.

References

1. Velagaleti RS, Pencina MJ, Murabito JM, Wang TJ, Parikh NI, D'Agostino RB et al. Long-term trends in the incidence of heart failure after myocardial infarction. *Circulation* 2008;**118**:2057-62.

2. Orlic D, Kajstura J, Chimenti S, Jakoniuk I, Anderson SM, Li B et al. Bone marrow cells regenerate infarcted myocardium. *Nature* 2001;**410**:701-5.

3. Kocher AA, Schuster MD, Szabolcs MJ, Takuma S, Burkhoff D, Wang J et al. Neovascularization of ischemic myocardium by human bone-marrow-derived angioblasts prevents cardiomyocyte apoptosis, reduces remodeling and improves cardiac function. *Nat Med* 2001;**7**:430-6.

4. Kawamoto A, Gwon HC, Iwaguro H, Yamaguchi JI, Uchida S, Masuda H et al. Therapeutic potential of ex vivo expanded endothelial progenitor cells for myocardial ischemia. *Circulation* 2001;**103**:634-7.

5. Mangi AA, Noiseux N, Kong D, He H, Rezvani M, Ingwall JS et al. Mesenchymal stem cells modified with Akt prevent remodeling and restore performance of infarcted hearts. *Nat Med* 2003;**9**:1195-201.

6. Schachinger V, Erbs S, Elsasser A, Haberbosch W, Hambrecht R, Holschermann H et al. Intracoronary bone marrow-derived progenitor cells in acute myocardial infarction. *N Engl J Med* 2006;**355**:1210-21.

7. Lunde K, Solheim S, Aakhus S, Arnesen H, Abdelnoor M, Egeland T et al. Intracoronary injection of mononuclear bone marrow cells in acute myocardial infarction. *N Engl J Med* 2006;**355**:1199-209.

8. Penicka M, Widimsky P, Kobylka P, Kozak T and Lang O. Images in cardiovascular medicine. Early tissue distribution of bone marrow mononuclear cells after transcoronary transplantation in a patient with acute myocardial infarction. *Circulation* 2005;**112**:e63-5.

9. Geng YJ. Molecular mechanisms for cardiovascular stem cell apoptosis and growth in the hearts with atherosclerotic coronary disease and ischemic heart failure. *Ann N Y Acad Sci* 2003;**1010**:687-97.

10. Wollert KC, Meyer GP, Lotz J, Ringes-Lichtenberg S, Lippolt P, Breidenbach C et al. Intracoronary autologous bone-marrow cell transfer after myocardial infarction: the BOOST randomised controlled clinical trial. *Lancet* 2004;**364**:141-8.

11 Meyer GP, Wollert KC, Lotz J, Steffens J, Lippolt P, Fichtner S et al. Intracoronary bone marrow cell transfer after myocardial infarction: eighteen months' follow-up data from the randomized, controlled BOOST (BOne marrOw transfer to enhance ST-elevation infarct regeneration) trial. *Circulation* 2006;**113**:1287-94.

12 Meyer GP, Wollert KC, Lotz J, Pirr J, Rager U, Lippolt P et al. Intracoronary bone marrow cell transfer after myocardial infarction: 5-year follow-up from the randomized-controlled BOOST trial. *Eur Heart J* 2009;**30**:2978-84.

13 Sun L, Zhang T, Lan X and Du G. Effects of stem cell therapy on left ventricular remodeling after acute myocardial infarction: a meta-analysis. *Clin Cardiol* 2010;**33**:296-302.

14 Martin-Rendon E, Brunskill S, Doree C, Hyde C, Watt S, Mathur A et al. Stem cell treatment for acute myocardial infarction. *Cochrane Database Syst Rev* 2008:CD006536.

15 Thum T, Bauersachs J, Poole-Wilson PA, Volk HD and Anker SD. The dying stem cell hypothesis: immune modulation as a novel mechanism for progenitor cell therapy in cardiac muscle. *J Am Coll Cardiol* 2005;**46**:1799-802.

16 Schachinger V, Assmus B, Britten MB, Honold J, Lehmann R, Teupe C et al. Transplantation of progenitor cells and regeneration enhancement in acute myocardial infarction: final one-year results of the TOPCARE-AMI Trial. *J Am Coll Cardiol* 2004;**44**:1690-9.

17 Stamm C, Westphal B, Kleine HD, Petzsch M, Kittner C, Klinge H et al. Autologous bone-marrow stem-cell transplantation for myocardial regeneration. *Lancet* 2003;**361**:45-6.

18 von Harsdorf R, Poole-Wilson PA and Dietz R. Regenerative capacity of the myocardium: implications for treatment of heart failure. *Lancet* 2004;**363**:1306-13.

19 Fadok VA, Bratton DL, Konowal A, Freed PW, Westcott JY and Henson PM. Macrophages that have ingested apoptotic cells in vitro inhibit proinflammatory cytokine production through autocrine/paracrine mechanisms involving TGF-beta, PGE2, and PAF. *J Clin Invest* 1998;**101**:890-8.

20 Hoffmann PR, Kench JA, Vondracek A, Kruk E, Daleke DL, Jordan M et al. Interaction between phosphatidylserine and the phosphatidylserine receptor inhibits immune responses in vivo. *J Immunol* 2005;**174**:1393-404.

21 Golpon HA, Fadok VA, Taraseviciene-Stewart L, Scerbavicius R, Sauer C, Welte T et al. Life after corpse engulfment: phagocytosis of apoptotic cells leads to VEGF secretion and cell growth. *FASEB J* 2004;**18**:1716-8.

22 Ankersmit HJ, Hoetzenecker K, Dietl W, Soleiman A, Horvat R, Wolfsberger M et al. Irradiated cultured apoptotic peripheral blood mononuclear cells regenerate infarcted myocardium. *Eur J Clin Invest* 2009;**39**:445-56.

23 Kim KL, Meng Y, Kim JY, Baek EJ and Suh W. Direct and Differential Effects of Stem Cell Factor on the Neovascularization Activity of Endothelial Progenitor Cells. *Cardiovasc Res* 2011.

24 Sandstedt J, Jonsson M, Lindahl A, Jeppsson A and Asp J. C-kit+ CD45- cells found in the adult human heart represent a population of endothelial progenitor cells. *Basic Res Cardiol* 2010;**105**:545-56.

25 Rustemeyer P, Wittkowski W, Jurk K and Koller A. Optimized flow cytometric analysis of endothelial progenitor cells in peripheral blood. *J Immunoassay Immunochem* 2006;**27**:77-88.

26 Gnecchi M, He H, Liang OD, Melo LG, Morello F, Mu H et al. Paracrine action accounts for marked protection of ischemic heart by Akt-modified mesenchymal stem cells. *Nat Med* 2005;**11**:367-8.

27 Mirotsou M, Zhang Z, Deb A, Zhang L, Gnecchi M, Noiseux N et al. Secreted frizzled related protein 2 (Sfrp2) is the key Akt-mesenchymal stem cell-released paracrine factor mediating myocardial survival and repair. *Proc Natl Acad Sci U S A* 2007;**104**:1643-8.

28 Gnecchi M and Melo LG. Bone marrow-derived mesenchymal stem cells: isolation, expansion, characterization, viral transduction, and production of conditioned medium. *Methods Mol Biol* 2009;**482**:281-94.

29 Gnecchi M, Zhang Z, Ni A and Dzau VJ. Paracrine mechanisms in adult stem cell signaling and therapy. *Circ Res* 2008;**103**:1204-19.

30 Mirotsou M, Jayawardena TM, Schmeckpeper J, Gnecchi M and Dzau VJ. Paracrine mechanisms of stem cell reparative and regenerative actions in the heart. *J Mol Cell Cardiol* 2011;**50**:280-9.

31 Korf-Klingebiel M, Kempf T, Sauer T, Brinkmann E, Fischer P, Meyer GP et al. Bone marrow cells are a rich source of growth factors and cytokines: implications for cell therapy trials after myocardial infarction. *Eur Heart J* 2008;**29**:2851-8.

32 Yang Z, von Ballmoos MW, Faessler D, Voelzmann J, Ortmann J, Diehm N et al. Paracrine factors secreted by endothelial progenitor cells prevent oxidative stress-induced apoptosis of mature endothelial cells. *Atherosclerosis* 2010;**211**:103-9.

33 Di Santo S, Yang Z, Wyler von Ballmoos M, Voelzmann J, Diehm N, Baumgartner I et al. Novel cell-free strategy for therapeutic angiogenesis: in vitro generated conditioned medium can replace progenitor cell transplantation. *PLoS One* 2009;**4**:e5643.

34 Lichtenauer M, Mildner M, Baumgartner A, Hasun M, Werba G, Beer L et al. Intravenous and intramyocardial injection of apoptotic white blood cell suspensions prevents ventricular remodelling by increasing elastin expression in cardiac scar tissue after myocardial infarction. *Basic Res Cardiol* 2011;**106**:645-55.

35 Trescher K, Bernecker O, Fellner B, Gyongyosi M, Schafer R, Aharinejad S et al. Inflammation and postinfarct remodeling: overexpression of IkappaB prevents ventricular dilation via increasing TIMP levels. *Cardiovasc Res* 2006;**69**:746-54.

36 Pfeffer MA, Pfeffer JM, Fishbein MC, Fletcher PJ, Spadaro J, Kloner RA et al. Myocardial infarct size and ventricular function in rats. *Circ Res* 1979;**44**:503-12.

37 Kadl A, Huber J, Gruber F, Bochkov VN, Binder BR and Leitinger N. Analysis of inflammatory gene induction by oxidized phospholipids in vivo by quantitative real-time RT-PCR in comparison with effects of LPS. *Vascul Pharmacol* 2002;**38**:219-27.

38 Pfaffl MW. A new mathematical model for relative quantification in real-time RT-PCR. *Nucleic Acids Res* 2001;**29**:e45.

39 Lichtenauer M, Mildner M, Hoetzenecker K, Zimmermann M, Podesser BK, Sipos W et al. Secretome of apoptotic peripheral blood cells confers cytoprotection to cardiomyocytes and inhibits tissue remodelling after acute myocardial infarction: a preclinical study. *Basic Research in Cardiology* 2011;**(in press)**.

40 Davis DR, Zhang Y, Smith RR, Cheng K, Terrovitis J, Malliaras K et al. Validation of the cardiosphere method to culture cardiac progenitor cells from myocardial tissue. *PLoS One* 2009;**4**:e7195.

41 Warejcka DJ, Harvey R, Taylor BJ, Young HE and Lucas PA. A population of cells isolated from rat heart capable of differentiating into several mesodermal phenotypes. *J Surg Res* 1996;**62**:233-42.

42 Gyongyosi M, Hemetsberger R, Posa A, Charwat S, Pavo N, Petnehazy O et al. Hypoxia-inducible factor 1-alpha release after intracoronary versus intramyocardial stem cell therapy in myocardial infarction. *J Cardiovasc Transl Res* 2010;**3**:114-21.

43 Gyongyosi M, Posa A, Pavo N, Hemetsberger R, Kvakan H, Steiner-Boker S et al. Differential effect of ischaemic preconditioning on mobilisation and recruitment of haematopoietic and mesenchymal stem cells in porcine myocardial ischaemia-reperfusion. *Thromb Haemost* 2010;**104**:376-84.

44 Krombach GA, Kinzel S, Mahnken AH, Gunther RW and Buecker A. Minimally invasive close-chest method for creating reperfused or occlusive myocardial infarction in swine. *Invest Radiol* 2005;**40**:14-8.

45 Ortiz-Perez JT, Meyers SN, Lee DC, Kansal P, Klocke FJ, Holly TA *et al*. Angiographic estimates of myocardium at risk during acute myocardial infarction: validation study using cardiac magnetic resonance imaging. *Eur Heart J* 2007;**28**:1750-8.

46 Gyongyosi M, Blanco J, Marian T, Tron L, Petnehazy O, Petrasi Z *et al*. Serial noninvasive in vivo positron emission tomographic tracking of percutaneously intramyocardially injected autologous porcine mesenchymal stem cells modified for transgene reporter gene expression. *Circ Cardiovasc Imaging* 2008;**1**:94-103.

47 Sun N, Meng Q and Tian A. Expressions of the anti-apoptotic genes Bag-1 and Bcl-2 in colon cancer and their relationship. *Am J Surg* 2010;**200**:341-5.

48 Hanson CJ, Bootman MD, Distelhorst CW, Maraldi T and Roderick HL. The cellular concentration of Bcl-2 determines its pro- or anti-apoptotic effect. *Cell Calcium* 2008;**44**:243-58.

49 Cao J, Zhu T, Lu L, Geng L, Wang L, Zhang Q *et al*. Estrogen induces cardioprotection in male C57BL/6J mice after acute myocardial infarction via decreased activity of matrix metalloproteinase-9 and increased Akt-Bcl-2 anti-apoptotic signaling. *Int J Mol Med* 2011;**28**:231-7.

50 Ha T, Hu Y, Liu L, Lu C, McMullen JR, Kelley J *et al*. TLR2 ligands induce cardioprotection against ischaemia/reperfusion injury through a PI3K/Akt-dependent mechanism. *Cardiovasc Res* 2010;**87**:694-703.

51 Lazou A, Iliodromitis EK, Cieslak D, Voskarides K, Mousikos S, Bofilis E *et al*. Ischemic but not mechanical preconditioning attenuates ischemia/reperfusion induced myocardial apoptosis in anaesthetized rabbits: the role of Bcl-2 family proteins and ERK1/2. *Apoptosis* 2006;**11**:2195-204.

52 Darling CE, Jiang R, Maynard M, Whittaker P, Vinten-Johansen J and Przyklenk K. Postconditioning via stuttering reperfusion limits myocardial infarct size in rabbit hearts: role of ERK1/2. *Am J Physiol Heart Circ Physiol* 2005;**289**:H1618-26.

53 Marais E, Genade S and Lochner A. CREB activation and ischaemic preconditioning. *Cardiovasc Drugs Ther* 2008;**22**:3-17.

54 Li C, Tian J, Li G, Jiang W, Xing Y, Hou J *et al*. Asperosaponin VI protects cardiac myocytes from hypoxia-induced apoptosis via activation of the PI3K/Akt and CREB pathways. *Eur J Pharmacol* 2010;**649**:100-7.

55 Lu XY, Chen L, Cai XL and Yang HT. Overexpression of heat shock protein 27 protects against ischaemia/reperfusion-induced cardiac dysfunction via stabilization of troponin I and T. *Cardiovasc Res* 2008;**79**:500-8.

56 Efthymiou CA, Mocanu MM, de Belleroche J, Wells DJ, Latchmann DS and Yellon DM. Heat shock protein 27 protects the heart against myocardial infarction. *Basic Res Cardiol* 2004;**99**:392-4.

57 Conn KJ, Rich CB, Jensen DE, Fontanilla MR, Bashir MM, Rosenbloom J *et al*. Insulin-like growth factor-I regulates transcription of the elastin gene through a putative retinoblastoma control element. A role for Sp3 acting as a repressor of elastin gene transcription. *J Biol Chem* 1996;**271**:28853-60.

58 Kothapalli CR and Ramamurthi A. Benefits of concurrent delivery of hyaluronan and IGF-1 cues to regeneration of crosslinked elastin matrices by adult rat vascular cells. *J Tissue Eng Regen Med* 2008;**2**:106-16.

59 Matthews KG, Devlin GP, Conaglen JV, Stuart SP, Mervyn Aitken W and Bass JJ. Changes in IGFs in cardiac tissue following myocardial infarction. *J Endocrinol* 1999;**163**:433-45.

60 Virag JA, Rolle ML, Reece J, Hardouin S, Feigl EO and Murry CE. Fibroblast growth factor-2 regulates myocardial infarct repair: effects on cell proliferation, scar contraction, and ventricular function. *Am J Pathol* 2007;**171**:1431-40.

61 Wolfe BL, Rich CB, Goud HD, Terpstra AJ, Bashir M, Rosenbloom J *et al*. Insulin-like growth factor-I regulates transcription of the elastin gene. *J Biol Chem* 1993;**268**:12418-26.

62 Mizuno T, Yau TM, Weisel RD, Kiani CG and Li RK. Elastin stabilizes an infarct and preserves ventricular function. *Circulation* 2005;**112**:I81-8.

63 Mizuno T, Mickle DA, Kiani CG and Li RK. Overexpression of elastin fragments in infarcted myocardium attenuates scar expansion and heart dysfunction. *Am J Physiol Heart Circ Physiol* 2005;**288**:H2819-27.

64 Breivik L, Helgeland E, Aarnes EK, Mrdalj J and Jonassen AK. Remote postconditioning by humoral factors in effluent from ischemic preconditioned rat hearts is mediated via PI3K/Akt-dependent cell-survival signaling at reperfusion. *Basic Res Cardiol* 2011;**106**:135-45.

65 Hausenloy DJ and Yellon DM. Reperfusion injury salvage kinase signalling: taking a RISK for cardioprotection. *Heart Fail Rev* 2007;**12**:217-34.

66 Van de Werf F, Bax J, Betriu A, Blomstrom-Lundqvist C, Crea F, Falk V *et al*. Management of acute myocardial infarction in patients presenting with persistent ST-segment elevation: the Task Force on the Management of ST-Segment Elevation Acute Myocardial Infarction of the European Society of Cardiology. *Eur Heart J* 2008;**29**:2909-45.

67 Antman EM, Hand M, Armstrong PW, Bates ER, Green LA, Halasyamani LK et al. 2007 focused update of the ACC/AHA 2004 guidelines for the management of patients with ST-elevation myocardial infarction: a report of the American College of Cardiology/American Heart Association Task Force on Practice Guidelines. *J Am Coll Cardiol* 2008;**51**:210-47.

68 Hooper JA. Intravenous immunoglobulins: evolution of commercial IVIG preparations. *Immunol Allergy Clin North Am* 2008;**28**:765-78, viii.

69 Stangel M and Pul R. Basic principles of intravenous immunoglobulin (IVIg) treatment. *J Neurol* 2006;**253 Suppl 5**:V18-24.

70 Spahn DR, Cerny V, Coats TJ, Duranteau J, Fernandez-Mondejar E, Gordini G et al. Management of bleeding following major trauma: a European guideline. *Crit Care* 2007;**11**:R17.

71 Practice Guidelines for blood component therapy: A report by the American Society of Anesthesiologists Task Force on Blood Component Therapy. *Anesthesiology* 1996;**84**:732-47.

72 Contreras M, Ala FA, Greaves M, Jones J, Levin M, Machin SJ et al. Guidelines for the use of fresh frozen plasma. British Committee for Standards in Haematology, Working Party of the Blood Transfusion Task Force. *Transfus Med* 1992;**2**:57-63.

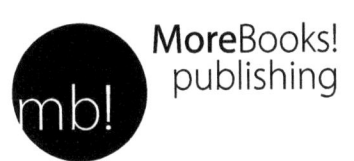

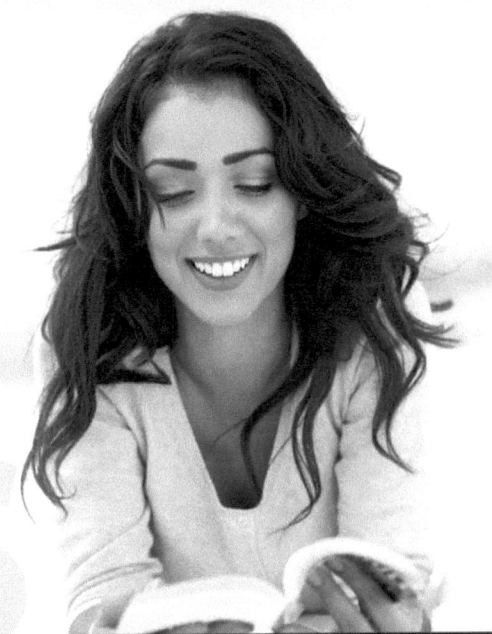

i want morebooks!

Buy your books fast and straightforward online - at one of world's fastest growing online book stores! Environmentally sound due to Print-on-Demand technologies.

Buy your books online at
www.get-morebooks.com

Kaufen Sie Ihre Bücher schnell und unkompliziert online – auf einer der am schnellsten wachsenden Buchhandelsplattformen weltweit! Dank Print-On-Demand umwelt- und ressourcenschonend produziert.

Bücher schneller online kaufen
www.morebooks.de

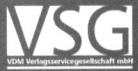

VDM Verlagsservicegesellschaft mbH
Heinrich-Böcking-Str. 6-8   Telefon: +49 681 3720 174   info@vdm-vsg.de
D - 66121 Saarbrücken   Telefax: +49 681 3720 1749 www.vdm-vsg.de

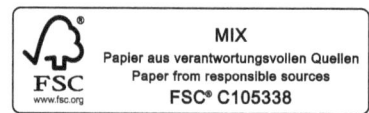

Printed by Books on Demand GmbH, Norderstedt / Germany